PRAISE FOR

"Stephen writes from the heart in a manner that is at the same time generous and filled with the reality of what it is like living with, through and after childhood cancer. A book filled with gentleness, compassion, hope and love. Onwards We Go is a book for everyone."

    - **DR. CARON STRAHLENDORF** B.C. Children's Hospital, Clinical Associate Professor, Head of Division of Hematology and Oncology, Department of Pediatrics, University of British Columbia

"As CEO for Ronald McDonald House BC & Yukon, I see families in similar situations on a daily basis, and by Stephen sharing his experience and emotions, and the reality of treatment for Jasper and how it affected both he and Barb, it is a reality check that those reading will relate to, whether they have experienced a cancer journey or not. It is a powerful and emotional story, which is real and is so impactful. Knowing Jasper was a gift and his joy and passion will stay with me always... onward."

    - **RICHARD PASS** Chief Executive Officer, Ronald McDonald House British Columbia & Yukon

"Parents of children with serious illnesses face a challenging journey. We are fortunate in British Columbia to have exceptional places of care and a support community for families. For more than thirty years the Canucks for Kids Fund has supported organizations like the BC Children's Hospital Foundation, Canuck Place Children's Hospice and Ronald McDonald House, so that families like the Mohans receive the care they need in BC. Thank you Stephen for sharing Jasper's story."

    - **TREVOR LINDEN** President of Hockey Operations, Vancouver Canucks

ONWARDS WE GO

a memoir by

STEPHEN MOHAN

ABOMINABLE
MOHAN
PUBLISHING

Onwards We Go

Copyright © 2017 by Stephen Mohan

All rights reserved. No part of this publication may be reproduced, distributed, or transmitted in any form or by any means, including photocopying, recording, digital scanning, or other electronic or mechanical methods, without the prior written permission of the publisher.

Published 2017

ABOMINABLE MOHAN PUBLISHING
British Columbia, Canada
mail@onwardswego.ca

ISBN 978-1-7750950-0-2

Cover photo by Barbra Mohan

Cover logos and registered trademarks are property of the Canuck Place Children's Hospice, the BC Children's Hospital and McDonald's Corporation and its affiliates.

A portion of the net proceeds of every book sale will be donated to the following institutions, each of which played a significant role in our journey:

Ronald McDonald House British Columbia
Canuck Place Children's Hospice
BC Children's Hospital

for the indomitable children and teens of the oncology ward: the undaunted Superheroes, the courageous Warriors, the most valiant of Knights, the toughest of Prizefighters, and the beautiful brave Princesses

for Barb, who has seen circumstances no mother should ever have to bear

and for Jasper

Contents

It's A Magical World   1
Monocularity   5
Pine Valley   9
Grasshopper   21
Trop Vite De Vivre - Trop Jeune De Mourire   25
A Taste Of Offshore Sailing   39
The Calamity Kid   57
Nutmeg Milkshakes   63
Yogurt & Coffee Beans   73
Jasper Solo   93
Carlotta   101
Low Blow To The Gut   133
Into The Fire   137
Onwards We Go...   143
Pray For Platelets   149
The Chemo Circus   161
A Miracle   171
Welcome Home   181
It's Raining Again   189
Picture Yourself On A Battlefront   203
Downwards We Go?   209
The Days Are Just Packed   213
Onwards He Goes   221
Weightless   225
House Full Of Empty Rooms   229
I Like To Ride My Bicycle   235
Breaking The Chains   253
I Think I Miss You Even More   271
Acknowledgements   277

PROLOGUE

IT'S A MAGICAL WORLD

I watch my twelve-year-old son through the kitchen window of the old house. He's playing alone outside. The rocky beach is one hundred yards away. He has navigated his way past the boardwalk and the dock, along the shoreline of rocks, and over the rusted, broken-down railroad tracks, the same iron tracks that used to haul the cradled wooden fish boats ashore on this small island in British Columbia. He pulls himself up on the end of a long creosote beam and carefully puts one small rubber boot in front of the other, like a tightrope walker at a circus. He uses his homemade driftwood sword for balance. Then he does a dramatic leap off the opposite end into the coarse shell sand and immediately goes into a run up the adjacent rocks.

He makes his way past the narrow gap that separates our island from the mainland at high tide. It's high tide now and there's a good wind blowing, making large enough waves to send a small spray up off the rocks. He makes a beeline to the water's edge and pauses, just standing there, losing himself in his thoughts to the suck and pull and swish before him.

Even from this long distance I can feel that mesmerizing sense he's experiencing. Growing up I had the same freedom to roam outside – to be immersed in my own imaginary world. Like him, I'd come across something so entrancing it would break the spell of whatever game I was playing: maybe an odd-shaped cloud passing against a clear blue sky, or a swath of tall pine trees swaying back and forth in a strong wind. Now here was my own son, so fortunate to have the freedom to chase dragons and command soldiers on his own piece of free earth, yet he too is awakened, in awe of wind and waves and the smells of the sea.

I think to myself: I am so blessed. I have everything a man could ask for. I have a loving wife and a beautiful son. I have a safe warm place to live. I've found true happiness. I actually mouth the words: "My life is perfect."

I'm broken out of my trance by the smell of lunch being overcooked. Time to call him inside before he disappears around the point. I open the creaky door and I'm hit with a whirled backdraft of chimney smoke coming over the roof. It's chilly outside. The boughs of the nearby red cedar trees are pumping up and down in the wind. Their branches are heavy with the weight of young cones ready to yield their pollen.

I ring the dinner bell at the top of the porch. Its clangs are carried away in a gust.

"Jasper! Lunch time!" I shout, but I doubt he can hear me anymore. I shield my eyes from the sun's glare off the water. He has moved directly into the light. I'm losing him.

An intense gust carries a cloud of smoke out to sea. A small branch from a nearby cedar falls to earth...

Jasper is just a silhouette now: a boy in a wool toque, a dark-colored winter jacket stuffed tightly inside a life-vest, with his clunky rubber boots, and his wooden sword ready in hand. He's all but a shadow against the shimmering diamond backdrop of the sea. He is disappearing around the point. He has gone beyond the reach of my calls. I strain to catch just one more glimpse of him, but I've lost him in the tumult of wind, wave, smoke and light.

CHAPTER ONE

MONOCULARITY

Wednesday, November 23, 2011, 10:00am

Jasper and Barb and I are at the B.C. Children's Hospital in Vancouver. Today was an appointment in the Oncology ward with Dr. Strahlendorf and Nurse Naomi. The news was not good. As I processed it, my surroundings began to reel and spin. The ground fell away from before me. I had to lie down. Right away. I'd never passed out before. "I'm going to pass out..." Too many sensations blasted me at once: the nauseating scent of hospital bleach cleaner, the overpowering bright fluorescent lights, the crinkling sound of the paper laid over the examination table as my body collapsed over it, and then the cold foreign glass of water pressed into my hand. I pulled deep breaths to keep the lights from going out. This couldn't be happening...

§

One day in 1972, when I was two years old, my mother found that my eyes gave a strange reflection. She took me to a doctor in Edmonton, Alberta where we lived. The doctor assured her that I was only experiencing some type of infection and that it would soon disappear. My mother refused to believe this diagnosis, and her persistence that it was something more than a simple infection convinced the doctor to conduct further tests. It was discovered that I had a cancer known as retinoblastoma in my left eye. Because of my mother's tenacity I was immediately slated for treatment. Unfortunately, in the 1970's retinoblastoma was still a rare form of cancer. I received horrible amounts of radiation treatment. They managed to save my right eye, but the cancer had spread too fast in my left, so it had to be removed. A glass orb was sewn in its place, and I continue to wear a prosthetic eye over that implant to this day. My right eye would remain intact and functional, but the heavy doses of radiation left me with a slight concave indentation to the temple on that side. The entire ordeal was a traumatic experience for my parents, and my infant self too.

Growing up, I didn't let my handicapped vision slow me down. In fact, most of the time I forgot about it altogether. Despite everyone telling me that I didn't have any depth perception, I rode bicycles, ski raced, played baseball, and took part in all of the activities that most young boys do. Sometimes I would see myself in a mirror and be reminded of the prosthesis. I'd wonder if it made me different in some form or another. Was I special? I couldn't help but wonder what it would be like if that other eye was still intact and functioning. How does everyone else view the world? Mom of course kept a baby album of me, and there are a couple of photos in there from before the cancer, when I still had a full range of vision. I'm a toddler, playing in the snow, looking back at the camera with two bright beautiful eyes. But I was far to young to remember what stereoscopic vision might be like.

As my body grew, every few years I would go through the tedious, several-days-long process of having a new prosthesis made and fitted. Usually I would get fair warning that I was due for a new one, as it would start to feel loose and sloppy in its socket. If it was too small it wouldn't stay seated properly and it would wander to a position in which it was staring off in some random direction – no doubt completely opposite of where my good eye was looking. This would leave me appearing more than just a little 'bat-shit crazy'. I couldn't tell when it wandered or spun around like that. I would come home from school and catch a surprising glimpse of myself in the bathroom mirror, "Oh *great*. How long has *that* been staring off at my nose?"

I lost my fake eye once during a school trip to the swimming pool. I did a backflip off a tire swing, and when I resurfaced I knew right away I was missing something important. One of my schoolmates announced very loudly that "Mohan's lost his eye!" and, of course, all the girls shrieked and fled the water. The boys thought this was a terrific opportunity and jumped in to be the first to find it. Yep, time for a new eye.

As I matured I often pondered what my overall lifespan would be as a result of previously having had cancer. Was I at any pronounced risk? Would I die early in life? Mom told me that I was in full remission and that I'd lead a 'normal' life, *but* I would be more susceptible to other forms of cancer in my future years. So I mostly put it out of my mind. I was blissfully unaware that I had overcome great odds and become a 'Survivor of Childhood Cancer'. I would go about experiencing as carefree a childhood as most other boys would.

CHAPTER TWO

PINE VALLEY

Friday, November 25, 2011 at 6:50am

The last few days have been a whirlwind. Jasper had headaches. Then the headaches were accompanied with vomiting, so we took him right away to the Emergency ward at the Powell River General Hospital. On Tuesday, he had a CT scan there. Wednesday: we arrived at the BC Children's Hospital and got the news from Dr. Strahlendorf that an anomaly has shown up on his brain. He got an MRI scan followed by a surgery - to relieve pressure on the brain and to take a biopsy. Thursday was recovery from surgery. It's Friday now and we are waiting for pathology of the biopsy, which will determine the next steps. The results will be in at 1pm today at the earliest.

§

My Dad ran away from his family in India. His father wanted him to go to law school. On the day of his convocation, for which his family thought he had travelled to Delhi, he actually left by steamer ship to England. When he became a British citizen, he wanted no trace of his past in India, so he dropped his old surname and used his first name, 'Mohan' in its place. They wanted to assign him an official first name, which he now did not have, so they simply filled out his papers for him as 'Man'. There was also some confusion at the time over Man Mohan's actual age. Back in India, he was too young to enter university, so he had to add some years to himself so he could attend. (In the future, whenever I asked Dad how old he was, he would just smile. I wonder if he himself even knew anymore.) England is where Man Mohan acquired his service papers and met my mother, Susan Kennedy. They fell in love, married, and immigrated to Edmonton, Alberta, Canada in the late 1960's.

They both found jobs with the Alberta provincial government, Susan as a secretary, and Mohan in a map-making department. With a decent job now acquired, Mohan chose to purchase his first car. He proudly showed his co-workers his new acquisition: a beautiful Volkswagen Karmann Ghia that he had bought from a used car lot. "Wow, Mohan - nice car. What did you pay for it?" they asked. He didn't understand. Of course he had paid what the sticker price on the window had advertised. The co-workers became aware that Mohan had not known he was supposed to 'haggle' for a deal on the car. He had been taken advantage of by the sales staff. Well, they weren't having any of that. They all marched down to the car lot, reprimanded the salesman for taking advantage of a newcomer to Canada, and got a large portion of Mohan's money back.

It was a casual working environment in that office. The other staff used to tease Mohan about how he wore a suit to work each day. He told them he felt it was important to look professional and give a good impression. Evidently, the suit worked, as it didn't take long for him to be promoted to a position as their supervisor, and in even less time he would graduate out of the map-making department altogether to an even higher posting in the workplace. He would eventually make a career with the Alberta Government and become an Assistant Deputy Minister for them.

I was born at the University of Alberta Hospital in Edmonton, on the first day of spring in 1970. My parents had bought a house in a new neighborhood of that city. My Dad was so excited the day I was born. Someone had told him it was a custom to hand out cigars in celebration of a new baby, so he proceeded to go door to door on his street. What he didn't realize was that everyone would invite him in for a drink. The neighbors were so accepting of him and his good news – even those who didn't know who he was. Despite Dad not being a drinker, or a smoker, he was invited inside to imbibe at several houses on the block. My mother was quite shocked to see the state he was in when he returned home later that afternoon.

Two years later I would be diagnosed with retinoblastoma. As anyone would imagine, Mom and Dad were worried and scared for me during my treatment. I was too young to remember anything of it. Eventually the disease was curtailed and I was given a status of remission. They breathed a sigh of relief when they could finally bring me home again from the hospital. On the day I came home there was a short fat boy riding a loud two-stroke mini-bike in the alley behind the house. He would ride past, a minute would go by, and then he would come back in the other direction – over and over... The din was akin to an airplane doing repeated fly-pasts. Dad wanted some peace and quiet so that I could fully rest. He marched out into the alley. Instead of raising his voice in aggression at the boy, he said with excitement, "Wow! That is a *very* nice motorbike you have there. *Very* nice. How about *you* take one more trip down the alley, and when you come back *I* will get a turn at riding this very fine motorbike?" Needless to say, the boy did not turn around and peace was again restored to the neighborhood.

Since their early days in Alberta, Mom and Dad had frequently escaped Edmonton for weekend trips to the Rocky Mountains. They kept a camping kit ready in the trunk of their car and on Friday afternoons they would depart straight from work to Jasper National Park. These trips fuelled their dream to live outside the city. They bought a three-acre heavily forested property forty kilometers southwest of Edmonton off of Pine Valley Road.

Dad would build a house on this property. He had long been a fan of the Western genre in books and films, in particular 'River of No Return', which was largely filmed in Alberta. This was his chance to build a chalet style, A-frame timber house. He found some plans in the back of an issue of 'Sunset' magazine. He knew absolutely nothing about building a house when he started it. The staff at the building supply store laughed at him when he asked what a 'two-by-four' was. Well, he would show them he was more than capable. Many might think it odd that a small East Indian man would have such wild western dreams. But consider all the English folks (like the Beatles) who flocked to India in search of an ashram. Dad set to work, undeterred by his inexperience or the sheer scope of the large project ahead of him.

For a while we lived in a tiny Boler trailer on the property while Dad built the house on weekends. Mom had given birth to a second baby boy. She was anxious about the completion of the new home with the prospect of this growing family. There was no water well on the property yet and she was getting tired of the long trek to fetch a bucket of water from the nearest neighboring house with my brother and I in tow. The Boler was clearly becoming too small for all of us. We were getting too big to be bathed in a garden pail. Dad built a rough 'cabin' for the interim winter months until the house was at a stage we could move in. In the end it turned out to be a fine home and, although I have distinct memories of the cedar shake roof leaking like a sieve during the summer rains, it proved to be a cozy and warm haven for the entirety of my childhood years. After we moved in Mom gave birth to another baby boy, and the five of us settled into an idyllic country life on the acreage.

Pine Valley was a fantastic place to grow up. Our property was situated between a turkey ranch and a chicken farm, so although we were forever losing dogs to the rifles of the farmers, it also meant we had vast areas of treed wilderness in which to roam. It was a massive area that included boggy swamps, forests of pine trees, wide-open prairie farmlands, sandy dunes, a shallow lake-like slough system, and a lush valley that the North Saskatchewan River flowed through. We could disappear all day with the other kids in the neighborhood. We would build elaborate tree forts, play war games, climb trees, and ride our bicycles down the endless dirt roads. We would spend days upon days constructing entire cities for our toy dinky-cars in the sandbank ditches of the road that passed by our property. Or we would fashion crude wooden weapons and go to battle against each other in the never-ending bush. We would build our own treehouses, and go-carts, and ramps to jump our bicycles off. A jar of nails and a hammer could keep us busy for weeks. Or even just a simple shovel. Sometimes we would go out in the bush and dig holes – massive holes – the kind you would have a hard time getting back out of – just because we could.

It was a tightknit community and the families in the area helped each other out. They rallied to each others' aid, whether it was digging a new well with shovels and buckets, rounding up an escaped pig, or mobilizing to plunder prime lumber spilled from an overturned semi-trailer that had descended too fast down the tight curvy road into the nearby river valley.

What a terrific place to raise children: without any boundaries and still relatively safe. I can only think of a couple times when our lives were actually in danger. Once, a bunch of us almost drowned when we fell through a crust of snow and ice that was hiding a septic field beneath. But we quickly learned from mistakes like that one – the message especially driven home by the accompanying putrid smell and vivid visual reminder of the contents of that field.

Mom would never be fully surprised when I returned home from experiences such as the septic field swim, or if I was covered in blood from falling out of a tree or the like. She had come to expect that there were bound to be lots of cuts and bruises due to the wild place we lived in.

Mom always made an effort to be involved in our lives. At different times she was a Cub Scout leader, Assistant School Librarian, School Secretary, and even a School Bus Driver. Many kids still remember travelling on her bus, coming home from school one winter day on the snowy country roads, when we hit a patch of ice at 80 km/h. The bus drifted sideways down into a snow filled ditch. The kids went deadly quiet and all eyes looked forward to see our fate. I think anyone else in that driver's seat would have resigned themselves to the fact we were headed into the abyss of a deep snow bank, and that there was nothing for it but to brace for impact. I think all the kids on the bus were expecting that same outcome. But not my Mom. She stomped that bus' gas pedal to the floor. It sent the roar of the engine through the roof. She countersteered us back onto the road, blowing a huge plume of snow skywards in the process. An eerie silence held for a couple of long seconds as everyone contemplated what had just happened. Then, all at once the entire bus erupted in cheers for Mom. I was so proud of her that day.

Mom was also an excellent seamstress and sewed a lot of our clothes; shirts, jackets, pajamas, pants, and Halloween costumes. My brothers and I would come home from our daily exploits in the back forty with torn knees in our pants. Mom would be kept busy sewing them back together with patches. Upon arrival home from our grubby endeavors, we would no doubt be absolutely filthy little creatures, covered head to toe in clouds of dirt. She made us strip off all our dirty clothes outside the house and then it was straight into the tub. Mom would run a hot bath for us heavily spiked with a bottle of 'Dettol', an antiseptic solution used for cleaning wounds. To this day I still associate the smell of Dettol with a hot bath.

Mom also introduced me to skiing, a sport that would become a true passion of mine. There was a Nordic ski club in the nearby town of Devon. Every winter, the club would set an immense network of cross-country ski trails in the North Saskatchewan River valley. Sometimes we would ski on these at night with the track brightly lit by the stars and moon above. There was also a downhill ski club in the river valley that shared the same chalet. The first time I watched the skiers whiz down the slopes I was intrigued. I herringboned my cross-country skis, one over the other, up the slope. Mom could see the sheer joy in my face as I careened back down toward her, barely in control. She knew right away that she had lost me to downhill skiing. I got hooked on that thrill of speed. She invested in some downhill specific equipment for me and I was enrolled in the Nancy Greene ski-racing league. I fell in love with the sport of racing slalom. Mom would come watch me on race days. She would tromp up the steep snow and ice covered slopes, and patiently stand waiting in the biting cold wind. Often it was colder than minus twenty degrees Celsius. Then, I would rush past her for all of three seconds and she would loudly cheer me on. She was so supportive of me.

When I was ten, Mom took me to a doctor for some issues I was having with a leaky bladder. It had to be rectified with an operation under anesthetic. The operation left me recovering in hospital for a full summer with a six-inch wide incision across my abdomen and a catheter inserted up my penis. Exiting the center of the incision were three clear tubes taped together, the largest one being half an inch in diameter. Just seeing these tubes snake out of the blankets and taped to the bed rail was akin to a horror movie for me. I couldn't bring myself to look at the actual incision site.

On the lighter side, I shared the room with three other bedridden boys of my age. We would tell jokes to each other, but oh, the mess of hosing coming out of my belly would hurt so much when it came to laughing at a punch line. I spent my time pouring over brochures of motorized go-carts and trikes. Mom said that she *might* consider me having one when I was finished in the hospital. Mom was always a bit hesitant about allowing me to have anything with a gas powered motor. Given my past track record this was probably wise on her part. I didn't end up with a go-cart, but I did manage to remove some serious amounts of skin from my backside while riding a friend's cart later that summer.

The time came for the tubes to be removed. I clearly remember the doctor hovering above me, answering my queries about whether this would hurt or not. "You may feel a slight tug. I will do it on the count of three. One... Two..." He pulled it out before reaching three. Whoa. Yes, it hurt. I felt so cheated that he had not pulled on the count of three. What a liar. He told me it was for the better, as I would have otherwise tensed up for it. Yeah - no kidding. And that was definitely not 'a slight tug.'

I also recall one night that I did not want to be left alone in that hospital. Mom had to go home to tend to my two brothers. I was very upset and simply *could not* be consoled. I was sobbing uncontrollably when she left the room. Years later Mom revealed to me that it broke her heart when she heard my prolonged call as the elevator doors closed in front of her: "Mooooooooommmmm..."

It was probably an unfair card to play on my part, because I knew very well that she couldn't stay. But I was a kid, felt cheated and lied to in this hospital, and did not want to be here – so I was letting it be known.

CHAPTER THREE

GRASSHOPPER

Friday, November 25, 2011 at 10:00pm

UPDATE: We have been discharged from the hospital for the weekend. THE PLAN: Monday morning will be an 8-hour surgery to remove the tumor. He will remain under anesthesia all of Tuesday during which he will have another MRI. Then he will recover in hospital for 5 to 8 days. The tumor is operable and the plan is for a 100% cure. Jasper is looking great and he is very strong, brave and positive. Barb and I look forward to a full nights sleep and a weekend away from the hospital as a family. We feel well supported from all of our family and friends.

§

My father was a very intelligent and wise man. I was proud to have him as my Dad. He loved me very much and told me often. He also told me he was proud of me, and would give me a warm embrace when doing so. I was his 'Grasshopper'.

My friends liked my Dad too. I think it was because he was so different – a short, brown, peaceful East Indian man with a foreign accent and a drive to do the abnormal (like travelling from India to build a timber house in Pine Valley). Some of my friends were too shy to approach him, because Dad could be mysteriously quiet. But occasionally one of my more engaging mates would show interest in some project or other that Dad was working on. Surprisingly, Dad would spring to life and treat us to a lengthy one-sided discussion in which he would become very animated and excited. Perhaps it was because he was so passionate about those topics; Amateur Radio, or the Kon-Tiki Expedition, or Transcendental Meditation, or badminton – these were strange subjects to any kid growing up on the prairies of Alberta.

Dad enjoyed tinkering with the internals of electronics. He had a bench dedicated to this art located in the dirt-floored basement of the house. To access this space you had to lift a large plywood trap door in front of the laundry machines. Then, you would descend a steep ladder. Below was dark, save for a single lamp lighting up the workbench. The visitor was met by a strong smell of solder smoke as Dad pulled apart all sorts of electronic devices and then reconstructed them into who-knows-what. There were bins full of sorted diodes and resistors and capacitors, all stacked high above the bench. Neatly piled circuit boards and spool upon spool of colored wire were everywhere. In the center of the bench would be the latest project: a transceiver or an oscilloscope, or a Teletype, or...? Ready at hand was the hot soldering iron, with a coil of tinned wire and a pot of flux beside it. All the while a Ham radio crackled away in the background with the occasional warbled voice of someone checking in from foreign lands. "sssssssszzz.....CQ, CQ, CQ... CQDX....sssssszzzzzz..." Prominently placed at the edge of the Ham radio was the mechanical Morse code Keyer, with its paddle ready to communicate "dits" and "dahs" across the world. Dad's amateur radio call sign was VE6AZM. The basement scene was quite a spectacle to behold. Friends couldn't help but ask, "Stephen, is your dad a spy?"

Dad would build gigantic elaborate Amateur Radio antennas behind our house. Eighty-foot high towers with quad beam spider-looking arrays perched atop, which he could send spinning 'round and 'round remotely from the house, pointing them in the direction of the signal he wished to capture.

On Saturdays, Dad would commandeer my brothers and I for a trip to the local garbage dump where we would rummage for 'new' parts. This was followed by a perusal of the nearby scrapyard where we would search for any 'useful' electronics that had been haphazardly tossed away by some unfortunate soul who didn't possess repair skills. Afterwards, it was down to the river to skip rocks and share some soda pops and a bag of glazed donuts.

One find at the dump was the shell of a discarded satellite dish. This inspired Dad to construct the necessary pieces to build a working satellite-television receiver. I remember the trial run of the system. He hooked up our television to a string of other devices he had cobbled together. My brothers and I, all between the years of twelve and fifteen, gathered eagerly around the television, which Dad had placed outside next to the dish. What a surprise when the first images appeared out of the static and revealed... the Playboy channel. That wasn't the first time I had heard him utter the words "Oh boy. You're mother is going to kill me..." in his light East Indian accent.

CHAPTER FOUR

TROP VITE DE VIVRE - TROP JEUNE DE MOURIRE

Monday, November 28, 2011 at 12:07pm

Change of plan. No surgery today. Professionals and specialists have been discussing Jasper's case all weekend. Chemo will be done first, then maybe surgery with radiation, or just radiation at a later date. We figure any day they tell you that you don't have to have brain surgery is a good day! Tests and a surgery for an access port in his chest will be carried out for the rest of the week. Chemo starts Friday. It'll be a strong chemo cocktail of 6 months duration. Out of the frying pan, into the fire.

§

My teenage years fell in the turbulent 1980's. As if it wasn't enough for a young mind to worry about the pressures of school, adolescence, and the arrival of the

Cold War... Mom developed breast cancer. I was worried that she was going to die. She had a mastectomy and then chemotherapy. It was pretty hard on her. She lost her hair during chemo. I remember so many silk scarves draped across her bedroom chest-of-drawers. As a teenager I didn't handle it well, and at the time the thing to do was largely ignore it and 'keep a stiff upper lip' about the entire matter.

I think it was a combination of not talking about the disease and the worry I was experiencing of possibly losing my mother that lead me to rebel a bit and distance myself emotionally from her. On top of that, we had just sold the acreage house and moved into the nearby town of Devon. I suppose it had made sense to move into town. Mom was constantly driving back and forth for our extra curricular activities, groceries, her job, and our schools. Mom and my brothers made a convincing argument that they wanted to be in town and Dad was ultimately swayed. I hated living in Devon. It was a pimple of an oil town on the face of a flat scraped prairie landscape. I missed our acreage, and the uniqueness of the home Dad had built for us there. My dog 'Poochie', a white Samoyed with a black fur patch over one eye, had spent the previous ten years roaming free on that property. Now she was limited to a suburban backyard. I felt the same confines as Poochie. Sadly, she died a month after we moved. To me, it was like an omen that we shouldn't have moved into town.

So, I rebelled. It was typical teenage stuff – loud music, excessive drinking, speeding, dabbling in 'pharmaceuticals', and spending my time away from home looking for trouble. Most of this was done with some like-minded trouble-seeking cases: we got dubbed 'The Ratt Pack", Ratt being an 80's hair band that we used as our partying, devil-may-care lifestyle role models. 'Trop vite de vivre – trop jeune de mourire' was scrawled on the lead guitarist's electric axe, and I openly embraced the mantra. Jokingly, I made a plan to kill myself on a future birthday by fully tattooing every inch of my skin and riding a chopper motorcycle over a cliff in the desert; all with my hair lit on fire and accompanied by a deafening soundtrack of heavy metal music. I'm happy to report that prophecy wasn't fulfilled.

One healthy form of escape I found was bicycling. I bought a road bike and began riding it like a fiend. My best friend Robbie and I dabbled a bit in some racing. We watched far too many cycling movies together. Somehow we came to the conclusion that cycling meant pounding out an eighty-mile ride and finishing it off with a heaping bowl of pasta in front of reruns of the Tour de France – then repeat.

I had always been drawn to individual sports versus team endeavors, and cycling was a great escape from my problems. I trained all day on the straight, flat, open prairie roads. I would listen to my Sony Walkman with my head down and simply tap away a rhythm on the pedals. This got me in trouble once when I wasn't fully paying attention to where I was going. Riding along at a good clip in a musical daze, I flipped face first into the open trunk of a parked car on the side of the highway. Miles and miles of prairie nothingness – who put that car there? It was stopped for a tire change. Boy, did I ever give the guy changing his front wheel a fright. I left that incident in an ambulance. My bike was demolished. My face was covered in stitches. I'd spend the rest of that summer on crutches.

If it involved going fast, I was interested. Robbie had got me into racing bicycles. Now the two of us would spend an entire summer building and racing GPV's (Gravity Powered Vehicles). I had discovered the idea in a *BMX Action* magazine. Essentially these were heavily modified BMX bicycles, but they no longer resembled anything close to a BMX by the time Robbie and I were finished building them. The frames were fully stripped of their parts - drivetrain and all. The drivetrain with its sprockets, cranks and chain was tossed aside. We didn't need them – these contraptions were gravity-powered. To start, I would flip the frame upside-down. Then, the front forks were reinstalled but were radically pre-bent to stick out directly in front of the bike. With the wheels back on, the combination of the swept fork and the inverted frame would make the bike ride very close to the ground. A seat tube and saddle were then suspended precariously over the rear wheel. The handlebars were swept as far forward and down as their mounts would allow – real 'knuckle draggers'. All of these modifications would result in a long low machine that looked fast just standing still. The rider would then lay face down stretched out flat on top of this speed sled. In this prone position I was ready to take flight. I'd be balanced in a tuck, my hands reaching far out in front of me, and my feet somewhere behind me on the pegs that projected out of the rear axle. I was an accident just waiting to happen.

The first test runs were down the steep paved road to the ski club chalet. Robbie and I were thinking it a wise choice, as there was little traffic and a nice long run-out at the bottom to slow us down. We needed that run-out because the first models didn't have brakes. Say a prayer and hope for the best before pushing off at the top of the road. Then it would be an all out gravity fed adrenalin high the entire plunge to the bottom. Was this dangerous? Yes, of course it was. So, for protection I would wear the padded ski equipment that I used for racing gates in the winter and my full-face ski helmet.

When we crashed it was catastrophic. On one descent I came into a turn way too hot. The bike skidded out from underneath me, repeatedly bouncing itself forty feet in the air before flinging its remains deep into the nearby treetops. Meanwhile I came to rest in a field of gravel - using my arm as a brake. I gathered up the pieces, made some makeshift ambulatory fixes to myself and limped home. Later I walked in the door of our house to Mom's remark of "Oh, no... what have you done *this* time?" She spent the rest of the evening picking the gravel out of my body with tweezers.

Survival requires evolution. Not wanting to remove ourselves from the gene pool just yet, Robbie and I fitted later models with brakes. By this time several other thrill seekers had joined us and we had a small squad racing together. Competition breeds experimentation, so we tried making the GPV's more streamlined. We built aerodynamic fairings out of wire and paper-mache. We started manufacturing our own disc wheels by stretching a wide roll of industrial grade plastic tape (a junkyard find of Dad's) over the expanse of the wheels. Anything that might make us go faster. Unfortunately many of these 'mods' didn't stand up to our destructive crashes.

On one of the bikes we added a speedometer and a banana seat. We would attempt to put two riders aboard. There was not much room on the banana seat, so a friend's little brother took up the position behind me. While the seat worked fine, the problem was this kid kept trying to look over my shoulder to read the speedometer. His weight shifts were causing me to lose control over our steering. "80-K an hour!" is the last thing I remember before waking in a ditch with my head buried to my shoulders in mud.

Soon we started seeking out the longer steeper roads in the area. There were some good ones in Edmonton that descended out of the downtown core into the river valley. The problem was the traffic. We would need someone to control the traffic at each intersection of our descent. We enlisted a few of our youngest brothers with some walkie-talkies. Picture a ten-year old walking into an intersection with his hand held upright, hailing cars to stop. Then, six helmeted teenagers wearing ski equipment scream through on disc wheeled machines that resemble something out of '*Tron*'. The little boy then nonchalantly walks back to the curb.

It seems a lot of my harebrained ideas included Robbie. We decided we would like to be rich, but we didn't want to work to get there. We wanted an 'easy' route to fortune. Surely panning for gold on the North Saskatchewan River would line our pockets with enough dollars to keep us in bicycles for the rest of our days? We liberated several hundred pounds of tools from Robbie's garage. We looked at a map and... No, we didn't even look at a map. And we didn't know the first thing about panning for gold either. We were just going to wing it. This was supposed to be easy, remember? We loaded pickaxes, shovels, rakes, and hoes onto our backs and started a slog upriver. That summer sun burning down on us was so intense. We were both packing in far too much of a load. At the end of a full day's hike we found a spot to hide our equipment. Good thing because we were both close to heat exhaustion. On our hike home we formed a plan to return with enough wooden boards, hammers and nails to build a sluice box to separate our gold nuggets from the river's chaff.

We never got rich. That could be because...we never went back. Somewhere out there under a large poplar tree is a cache of tools worth well over a thousand dollars. On future visits to Robbie's house I would cringe when his dad was looking for a garden implement. "Robbie! *Where* is my *shovel*?"

Robbie and I attended a small high school in Devon. There were about a hundred students in our graduating class, and that was the largest on record that the town had ever seen. Early on, there was pressure from the school to choose a career path. Guidance counselors told me I had to either pick physics, biology, or chemistry as a science to lead to any possible university options. I didn't know what future career to pursue, so I took all three. It was a bit of a mistake, as the course load was heavy enough that I didn't do well in any of them.

When Robbie and I were stuck in math class, we hatched a plan to someday be boat builders and live aboard our own grand sailboat in Vancouver harbor (a bit of a reach for two boys growing up on the prairies who had not sailed so much as a rubber duck). Those boring math classes were the perfect place to spawn that type of plan. I scratched a long trail of hash-lines on the wall next to my desk marking each passing day of agony. The teacher bred contempt. "Enjoy it while you got it 'cause it all goes downhill after forty", he told us. What a terrible attitude for a teacher of young minds. Most of the class laughed along with him, but it actually enflamed and inspired me to resist ending up like that poor sod. I'd prove him wrong, oh boy. This is something that continues to this day to fire me up. When someone says it can't be done, or it's unobtainable or a silly pursuit, or you're too old, it seems to kindle something in me to pursue it to my fullest to prove him or her wrong. I think I got this "Well, I'll show *you!*" attitude from my father.

I coasted through the rest of high school, with the school's principal, teachers, and guidance counselors constantly pushing the message on the students that "you will look back on these years as the best of your lives." Bull shit, I thought, getting out of high school will be like being released from jail.

In the winter seasons I worked as a Coach for the Devon Ski Club's Nancy Greene racing program. It was a lot of fun teaching kids aged five to thirteen to race gates. It was so satisfying showing these kids a technique and then seeing smiling faces of accomplishment beaming back at you. We always did well at the races. Plus, my team and I were a mischievous bunch, especially on trips to other clubs, or when we raced in the nearby Rocky Mountain resorts of Jasper and Banff. We were constantly being chased by the ski patrol for being up to no good. It was a lot of fun lightly corrupting young minds to fight the system. Of course, it was all harmless stuff; things like disobeying signs on the mountain, or cutting in line at the lifts, or hitting a big jump that was closed for use. What chance did a single ski patroller have against a pack of twenty kids (who could ski remarkably well) on a high speed bombing run straight through Jasper's Marmot Basin upper chalet 'SLOW' zone? Sometimes we got caught and heavily reprimanded. Then we'd go and do it again. What a bunch of troublemakers we were. When we were back in the town of Jasper, our reign of terror would continue; usually in the form of a travelling party, out on the streets of town with the teenagers of the team. "Cops!

Chuck yer' beers!" I was always the one that didn't hear the alarm raised, and on more than one occasion I found myself in the back of a police car.

I did a few late night shifts at the Devon Ski Club tending to the snow making guns. These guns fired water into the air and in the right temperatures it would fall as snow. The guns also had to be turned in a new direction every hour to spread the snow out over a large area. I recall one early morning when I found a ten-foot high solid ice mound in the middle of a run. The previous worker had fallen asleep during his shift. Hmmm… or was that me?

Occasionally I worked at the ski club as a 'Lifty', operating the club's rope tow lift. The rope tow was a loop of two-inch diameter line that stretched up to the far reaches of the hill and back down again. Skiers would hold onto the rope and be pulled to the top. An underpowered motor at the base of the hill accomplished this - barely. It was the lift attendant's job to shut down the machine if something went awry. There were lots of opportunities for this to happen. Rope tows are a good place to witness carnage. For the first time skier using the lift, I would give instructions to move up beside the rope, slowly and gently close your mittens around it, and enjoy the safe ride as it carries you up the hill. Invariably they would do the complete opposite of what they were told and fiercely grab the rope with a death grip strangle. This would propel them violently forward, face first with their skis splayed out behind them. You would think that they would then let go, but I guess human instinct is to hang on till the lights go out. I was constantly stopping and starting the lift due to accidents. Sometimes one skier would fall down and not get out of the path of the lift, causing a massive pile up of bodies. Again, you would think people would have the sense to let go of the rope and step to the side to avoid a collision. Nope. This rope tow also featured a challenging steep incline at the very top for the last hundred feet. Some people just didn't possess the required strength in their hands to grip the rope anymore by this point. Their strength would give out, sending the rope zipping through their tired hands, and they would slowly slide backwards, bumping into the skier coming up behind them, and the skier behind them, and so on, and so on. Now, even though there were bodies stacked five or six high, no one would let go of the rope. The underpowered motor would not be able to take the strain. If I didn't get to the emergency stop button in time the entire machine would be fried. If I only had a dollar for every time I had to yell "People! LET - GO - OF - THE - ROPE!" I much preferred running the club's snowmobile to orchestrating the frustrating gong show of the rope tow.

Immediately following high school I worked for a summer in an office of the Alberta Government. I had to achieve this job on my own merit, as Dad did not want to risk showing any sign of nepotism, even though the position couldn't be any farther away from what his job was. I was to be assigned to an accounting department in Forestry. No, I did not possess anything resembling accounting skills. I was in charge of adding up the grocery bills of the fire crews working the province's forest fires. I would sit all day with an adding machine doing sums. Oh, how tedious and boring. Later in life I adopted a mantra to live by: I don't queue up, and I don't do sums. I think that accounting office is where I subconsciously ruled out doing math ever again if I could avoid it.

Just as my parents did when they first started working for the Alberta government, I too began planning weekly escapes to the mountains. I bought Robbie's old brown VW Sirocco. I would use this as my ticket out of town, having it fueled and loaded for Friday afternoons, ready for a weekend of adventure with friends. In the summer season, we would use it to travel into the Rockies to Canmore for rock climbing, mountaineering, hiking, camping, and mountain biking. In the winter, we would make the five-hour drive to the Sunshine Village parking lot in Banff National Park; accelerator pinned, tunes cranked, beers cracked open, and the car a wasteland of crushed Pringles and junk food wrappers strewn about the ski equipment and camping gear. We would arrive late at night, spread out a blue tarp, and lay down in our sleeping bags for a few hours of sleep under the stars. In the morning we would awaken covered in a dusting of snow. We would then sit upright in our sleeping bags and brew up breakfast on our portable camp stoves. Skiers would shake their heads and smile as they navigated around us on their way to the chalet for a lift ticket.

As much as it was dull and boring, the accounting job did pay well, so after a season of forest fires I had enough savings to make a stab at backpacking my way around Europe. A month before my planned departure to foreign lands, I saw a job advertised by a company that was building a new highway between Devon and Edmonton. I figured a little extra cash in my pocket for my travels wouldn't hurt so I signed up. They drove a bunch of us out to the job site, far from anywhere, on the windswept prairies. This was a road paving crew. The supervisor pointed at a large steamroller. "You're operating that one." He told me I was to follow behind another steamroller, which in turn was following behind a machine and crew that was laying down fresh asphalt. I had never driven anything remotely like this, but I was game. It was huge. I started it up and took my place in line. "Hey, this isn't so bad," I thought. "Easy money." The fellow on the roller in front of me shouted back. He told me I had to push the red button on the console. Okay. The entire machine erupted in a loud rumbling din and rattled violently in all directions. My eyes shook in their sockets. My butt bounced on the seat. The noise sounded like my head was inside a washing machine full of nuts and bolts. Apparently this was the 'Vibrating Drum Roller'. Three hours later the fellow in front of me gave me the signal for lunch. Thank God, peace at last and a chance to stop shaking and have a bite to eat. It lasted all of two minutes. The angry foreman came racing past in his pickup truck and ordered us to get rolling again. Late in the day I disappointingly watched a car full of my friends wave at me as they headed to Edmonton for an evening of fun and frivolity. That night after the crew was shuttled back to town I explained that I would not be returning the next day. Despite the crew's pleas and flattering comments that I was 'a natural' at driving a steamroller, I could not be swayed. I had my eyes on traversing the cobblestone roads of Europe, not the asphalt slabs of Alberta.

I bade leave to friends and family and slung a backpack over my shoulder to go 'find myself' in Europe. I managed to see a fair bit of England and Europe, and I really enjoyed travelling, but after a few months I ran out of money. I tried to secure a job as a ski instructor in the Austrian Alps, but it was late summer and none of the chalets were hiring yet. I returned to London, invested my remaining shillings in beer, and flew home to Edmonton.

CHAPTER FIVE

A TASTE OF OFFSHORE SAILING

Friday, December 2, 2011 at 7:25am

Jasper has surgery this afternoon for a 'center line' - a port placed in his chest where chemo can be administered. They will also draw some spinal fluid for future stem cell work. Chemo will start Monday. He will have two protocols of chemo over the next 4 to 6 weeks and will be in hospital for that entire time. After that, neurosurgery may be necessary to remove the tumor, in combination with radiation treatment and a further 6 months of chemo. Jasper continues to smile thru last week's field of tests. Yesterday a PET scan came back with good results showing only the tumor in his brain - nowhere else in his body. That was a huge relief for us all. Barb and I are thankful for all our family and friends support through this. We are still managing to cope with it all. We take turns falling to pieces. Jasper is calling me his "Public Relations

> Manager". At this point I can't respond to each and every message - I just don't have the energy. I will continue to give everyone updates when I can.

Tuesday, December 6, 2011 at 9:09am

> Chemo started last night. His nausea is being kept in check so he may sleep a fair bit today as a result. Yesterday the spinal lumbar test came back with good results - there are no cancer cells anywhere else in his body. Also he got moved to a much nicer room with a window. And the Vancouver Canucks and the B.C. Lions visited him and that cheered him up.

§

My parents had always dreamt of living on the coast of British Columbia. Even our house back on the acreage had a map of Saltspring Island displayed prominently on a wall. They looked at purchasing a piece of property on that island, but ended up buying a small timber cabin outside of Qualicum Beach on Vancouver Island with the idea that they would retire early there. I had nothing holding me to Alberta, so I chose to follow them out to the coast. It was just before they left that I spied an ad in the classifieds of a west coast boating magazine about an outfit in B.C. that was providing ten-day sailing trips aboard a traditional tall ship. Coincidentally, our neighbor's daughter had just returned from one of these trips and was raving about her experience. It appealed to me greatly. It was right up my alley. Perhaps it could somehow also lead to my dream of building boats?

I plunked my money down for a voyage on the tall ship. I pointed the Sirocco towards the coast and never looked back. That summer I boarded the square topsail schooner *'Pacific Swift'* in Victoria and we sailed north to Desolation Sound, a beautiful area where the mountains come straight down into the sea. We worked as a group to sail the ship. We'd row the ship's boats ashore to play games and explore, and then returned to fresh baking and hearty meals aboard. The ship was run by 'The Sail and Life Training Society' (S.A.L.T.S.), an interdenominational Christian group. The crew was all so friendly and inviting. It was life changing. I was hooked.

When we returned to Victoria I was keen to stay involved with the *Pacific Swift* so I hung around the docks, living out of the Sirocco for a short period of time and couch-surfing when the opportunity presented itself. I'd be happy just to operate a broom if it meant I could somehow be involved with S.A.L.T.S. This was indeed looking like it could lead in the direction of my dream of building boats.

After several months of volunteering with the organization, I was invited to become one of the crew. Also, I would be the ship's caretaker when it was in port between trips. In the winter season I would work with a team preparing the ship for the next sailing season. Over time, I worked my way through various crew positions, such as Watch Leader, Boatswain's Mate, Watch Officer, and ship's Boatswain.

One requirement to be crew was that you had to be of Christian faith. Growing up I had not been overly involved with a church of any type. Apparently I'd been baptized as a baby. Mom would take me on Christmas Eve to the mass at the local Anglican Church. I would take Communion and sing the hymns there. Sure, I believed in God as I grew up. I prayed to him now and then. I had a certificate that said I had been baptized as a baby – that meant *something* to me. Church and Christianity certainly were not forced upon me in any serious way though. I guess you could call it 'Church: Lite'. Working with S.A.L.T.S introduced me to 'Church: Full-Strength'. My early days with S.A.L.T.S. involved a lot of personal inner exploration of my beliefs. I would go to the Bible studies and music jam sessions and the Sunday services with the S.A.L.T.S crew. Several of them had become close friends. They helped me reinvent my view of what a Christian was. Gone were my preconceptions of square, stuffy, Bible thumping, social misfits who go peddling door to door. These folks were hikers and mountain bikers, and they rode fast motorcycles, and could play a guitar with some edge to it. They went on exciting adventures. They weren't afraid of sharing. They were easy to talk to. They were so accepting of me. In short - they were cool. But I still couldn't figure how to say, "Yeah, I'm a Christian" with the same conviction that they did. Then one day I did just say it, was a little bit surprised at myself, and moved on. It was a bit of a non-event in the end – almost like others needed to hear me say it more than I needed to. At least I didn't feel any guilt or doubt that I couldn't work alongside the crew anymore. My Christian faith did grow strong, but without all the airy-fairy fluff of a Hallmark card or the sappiness of 'Kumbayah' around a campfire. My faith was borne from the wind and water and mountains that these tall ships were showing me.

It turns out that I had first laid eyes on the *Pacific Swift* many years before I had the opportunity to sail aboard her. I was sixteen and it was being built at the 1986 World Exposition in Vancouver. Every summer I would spend a couple of weeks at my Aunt's home in Sunset. From her house, the Expo '86 site was about a thirty-minute downhill coast on my BMX. The *'Swift* was being displayed as a working exhibit. It was in its final stages of construction under an open-air canopy and had staging wrapped around one side for the crowds to view the ongoing construction. Shipwrights were busy moving about on deck with overloaded tool belts on their hips. I remember the smell of fresh cut wood. The entire structure had a warm glow about it. I was completely oblivious to the important role this giant wooden cradle would later play in my life.

The *'Swift* would become my home under sail, voyaging all over the world. In 1990 the ship was to make the journey to the World Exposition in Seville, Spain. It would be almost a two-year voyage and I'd be aboard for a considerable portion of the trip. There was an empty berth available for its departure from Victoria. It was offered to me, after I'd shown so much enthusiasm for the coastal program. I would be the Boatswain's Mate and remain aboard until a crew change in Mexico.

The ship left Victoria with much fanfare and many speeches. The press was recording it all and families of the crewmembers filled the dock to capacity. We set sail off of Victoria and headed west. Our journey had finally begun. The following day we emerged from Juan De Fuca Strait into the wide-open Pacific Ocean. It was amazing being surrounded by the golden morning light of the sunrise and the fizzing sound of the slow heaving waves foaming past the hull around us. This was my first taste of offshore sailing. And what a taste it was: I spent the first hour of the day vomiting green bile. Dave, the ship's First Mate, and I climbed into the whisker shrouds under the bowsprit at the forward end of the ship. This was essentially a large net that we could sit in and have a clear uninhibited shot to projectile vomit into the sea. We would take turns throwing up, Dave and then I, but we would be laughing between convulsions, because we were in fact so happy to be finally sailing the ship out in the Pacific swell.

We sounded like the comic duo of Bob and Doug McKenzie.

"Beauty day, eh? Lookit' how different the color of the water is out here." Blechhh... Dave would empty his stomach contents through the whisker shrouds.

"Oh yeah, eh. She's a beaut alright." Blahhhh... I would dry-heave until my clenched abdomen muscles couldn't take any more. This we followed with the typical snorting fits of laughter that Bob Mckenzie was prone to. Then the cycle would repeat again. A couple a' 'hoseheads' – literally.

Our first port of call was to be San Francisco, so we had a long leg of sailing before us. It so happened that a smaller sailing schooner, the '*Alcyone*' of Port Townsend, was making the passage in our company. With only the horizon and the *Alcyone* to judge anything by, the size and effects of the ocean swell were put well into perspective. We would watch this eighty-one-foot long schooner and it's towering masts completely vanish behind the waves, only to reappear again moments later on the swell's next crescendo.

Arriving in a port city by tall ship definitely has some perks and advantages, and San Francisco and San Diego were no exceptions. We were usually moored close to a hub of activity. Maritime museums were keen to have us at their docks and would arrange for shore excursions for the entire crew. Sometimes this meant free tickets to an IMAX theater, a dinner event, or transportation in a van or bus. At times we were treated like rock stars, although we were content for the opportunity to have a cold pop, a hot shower, and a place to wash our laundry.

Once in Mexican waters, we made our first landfall outside of Ensenada. The ship had three rowing dories that were each capable of carrying a group of eight to ten crewmembers to shore. To maneuver the dory, four crewmembers would each take an oar under the command of a fifth person steering with a paddle in the stern. Everyone else would find a spot to sit amongst them. I took up the position of command in the stern and eight others climbed over the rail into the dory. As we rowed towards the shoreline I watched the two other dories from afar as they glided into the sandy beach. What I didn't see was that there was a pattern to the set of heavy breaking surf onto the beach. As we approached the shore I timed the waves completely wrong. The dory was taken up at a great speed by a big breaker. I was not ready for this, having never made a beach landing in surf before. I lost steerage altogether. The wave then skewed the dory sideways to the worst possible position. Everyone was thrown out as the boat rolled completely over. It disappeared briefly below the water and was then burped up from the sea onto the beach. Thankfully no one was seriously hurt, just some bumps and bruises – and my sore pride. I felt terrible. Everyone and their gear were completely soaked. There was beach sand in everything. Unfortunately, the dory itself was badly damaged, and although it served with the *Pacific Swift* for many years after, it would always bear the evidence of my poorly executed landing.

I really did enjoy travelling in Mexico. I seemed to fit in so well. Being partially of East Indian descent, I tan quite dark in the southern climates. I would often be mistaken as a local. Once, I was waiting in a line to use a telephone and even my own shipmates standing directly behind me didn't recognize me. Mexico was wonderfully cheap too, which was great for someone on a limited travel budget. I remember planting myself down beside a vendor who had a hibachi on the side of the road. He was grilling fresh fish for tacos. They smelled incredible. I sat there in the gutter for a long time eating one after another of those cheap delicious wonders. The tiny bottles of Coca Cola flowed as free as a mighty river - I practically burned a hole in my stomach guzzling back so many of them.

At this time the Baja peninsula was still a sleepy, laid-back locale. While many folks from the north had discovered it as a great vacation getaway spot, it was still devoid of the creeping box stores and retail chains of the western world. We sailed to the Coronado Islands, and explored the nothingness of rock outcrops and remote fishing villages. We visited the plastic and bone covered beaches of Bahia Tortuga. We made our way south to quiet Cabo San Lucas before sailing up inside the Sea of Cortes. We pointed the vessel south again to travel down the west coast of Mexico proper. I then flew home from Puerto Vallarta to Victoria to work for a season on the '*Robertson II*', a second tall ship in the S.A.L.T.S fleet.

The Swift's entire voyage was split into ten 'legs'. At the end of each leg some of the trainees, who had paid a fee to be there, left or joined the ship. Trainees were required to hold a high school diploma and be no older than twenty-five. Each trainee would be assigned a bunk, ladies up forward in the forecastle, and the young men in the center of the ship in the hold. The professional crew had their quarters in the aft portion of the ship. This included two Cooks, a Watch Officer, a Boatswain and Boatswain's Mate, the First Mate, and the Skipper in command. The trainees were required and expected to help sail and run the ship under the direction and tutelage of the professional crew – this was no holiday cruise with shuffleboard and cocktails on the Toledo deck. It took an entire crew to set sail, assist in meal preparations, raise the anchor, or launch the ship's dories. At scheduled points of the voyage the professional crew would also swap positions with a crew from home.

After a season of work at home, I had saved enough funds to purchase a berth as a trainee on the third leg of the voyage. This leg was to be a three month long circumnavigation of the Caribbean starting and ending in Miami. The Skipper and his wife (in the position of First Mate) were seasoned sailors of the Caribbean. They knew every nook and cranny, and some of the inhabitants as well, of these islands. We made landfall on all of the popular main islands and visited a high number of the out-of-the-way ones too. It was quite refreshing to be a trainee for a change, free to venture ashore and explore without the responsibility that accompanied being professional crew. I took advantage of this and adventured to the fullest extent I possibly could, searching out the little known destinations. I walked over a lava crust of the Soufriere volcano on St. Lucia (only learning afterwards that someone had fallen through it the week before and burned to death). I hiked into the clouds on the dicey trail to the peak of the Island of Nevis, where a misplaced step could be your last. I slept in a damp, aged stone fort in Nassau. I hitchhiked and rode bus-vans to remote bays for snorkeling. I swam naked in waterfalls deep in the jungle. I befriended stray dogs on sojourns up lonely mountain roads. I ate pamplemousse and bananas straight off the trees. I explored market places and danced to reggae and steel drum bands.

For the most part folks were welcoming and inviting to me. There was one exception when I was walking through a marketplace in Antigua with my friend Jim, the ship's Boatswain. Two young, tough locals were striding toward us through the crowd. As they passed by, one of them feigned a punch at my head. It being on my blind side, I never saw it happen and merely walked on by. Jim and I laughed about it afterwards. He told me of the disbelieving astonished looks on their faces because I hadn't flinched. Ya man, kool as a cucumber.

Horseracing is prominent in the Caribbean and I took the opportunity to watch some. Unlike most of the world who watch such events from the safety of their seats in a grandstand, the crowd here would stand three or four deep right up against the track railing. You could feel the flurry of wind as the horses galloped past. The thunderous sound of hooves meeting mud echoed through the ground up into your body. Being so close, I was almost swept up in a bad crash once. Down came a horse and jockey at full speed into a turn. Splinters of the track's white picket fencing were sent skyward and the spectators scrambled on top of each other to get clear. The mud and debris showered down around me. The horse and jockey returned to their feet unscathed, but many in the crowd were injured.

Although I escaped that incident unharmed, I did not fare so well from a motorcycle crash in the Dominican Republic. My fellow shipmate, Andrea, and I had rented a motorcycle and rode across the country, from Santa Domingo in the south to a remote northern beach. On the return trip I failed to see a trench across the road. The bike's front wheel hit it hard. Andrea and I went sailing through the air. Andrea landed somewhere behind me in my wake. I lost track of where the bike ended up.

I picked myself up and the delirium of shock set in immediately. We tried our best to make sense of our surroundings and plan our next move. Andrea's knee had a gaping cut, and I had blood streaming down my forearms. This road was in the middle of nowhere, surrounded by jungle. Now what? Dozens of locals appeared out of thin air. It seemed to happen so fast (perhaps due to the effects of shock?). No one spoke English. Andrea was lifted into the bed of a pickup truck. I struggled to lift myself up and over the tailgate. I realize the people meant well, but they then proceeded to lay the hot broken motorcycle down on top of us. The smell of gas and blood was nauseating.

We were driven hastily to a clinic in a small village where, by the time we arrived, it was nightfall. This clinic was a dark barren concrete building without any interior doors and there was no sign of any medical equipment about. Two armed policemen sat us down in a room devoid of anything but a table and chairs. A bright lamp swung from above. They proceeded to interrogate us in broken English. The officers did not appear to be happy at our responses, which were mostly borne out of our current state of shock and fear. We just wanted some medical attention. They wanted to know how much money we had. Were they asking for a bribe? It was so hard to understand their attempt at English. They wanted to see our passports. We didn't have them - they were stowed in a safe on the ship. This went on for what seemed an eternity.

Finally we were ushered into separate rooms for some 'treatment'. I was led into a poorly lit, dirty, cement space. There was one window and it was filled with the dozen or more faces of children pressed up against it, waiting for the show to begin. I was stripped down to my underwear and instructed to stand up with my arms out to each side. A doctor and nurse then took turns scrubbing and raking my entire body with a stiff dish brush and a bottle of straight iodine. To say it was painful would be an understatement. I don't think John Rambo had ever endured such torture. Andrea was not fairing any better in the room next door. She was worried, as nobody from the ship knew where we were or what had happened to us. Perhaps the police officers had understood our explanation, and contacted our ship? Also, her knee looked really bad. Andrea was concerned at the lack of cleanliness and low degree of medical expertise at hand.

There was now a new dilemma. Apparently the clinic had run out of thread to finish the suture to her knee. I was handed a piece of paper and, with a series of grunts and words I couldn't quite comprehend, was pushed out the door into the night. I made the most of the directions on the paper and ended up in a dark alleyway with a group of rough characters surrounding me. I had a fleeting thought that this could be my ultimate demise. I showed them the paper. They asked for money. I hesitated. With nothing to lose I gave them the only twenty US dollar bill I had. Again, a momentary thought – was I being robbed? The men guided me to a nearby warehouse. One of them went inside, there was some yelling, and when he emerged he pushed a paper bag of spooled suture thread into my hand. I did my best attempt at a limping run back to the clinic, my body throbbing everywhere under the duress of my wounds.

It is all a blur to me how we ever got back to the *Pacific Swift* late that night. I was so completely done in by then. I vaguely remember the car ride back and spilling out of a taxi onto the dock into the waiting arms of our shipmates.

The following day my friend Jim visited the motorcycle rental outfit and, after much haggling, paid for the damages to the bike. Unfortunately, Andrea's knee required further medical attention. With the possibility of gangrene setting in, she was flown back to North America for surgery. As for myself, I guiltily stayed with the ship. I experienced the temporary discomfort of my cuts and wounds for the next short while, but I continue to this day to bear the heavy shame of having played a key role in hurting Andrea and sending her home. There is a somewhat bright ending to this story. Her knee did eventually heal. She later went on to become the *University of British Columbia's Female Athlete of the Year*, and played for several years as Captain of the *Canada Women's National Soccer Team*.

When leg three was complete I was offered a place aboard as the boatswain's mate for the tour up the eastern seaboard of the United States, to Nova Scotia and Prince Edward Island, and then a transit up the St. Lawrence Seaway through Quebec City and Montreal, to finish in Kingston, Ontario. The hustle and bustle of the United States was definitely a wake up call after experiencing the laidback third world communities of the Caribbean.

And what a juxtaposition of culture it was. In Norfolk, Virginia I wandered into a rough neighborhood. A background symphony of police sirens hung constantly in the air. Business frontage was boarded up for blocks. Remnants of a once thriving community were barely detectable. It was like a 'Closed' sign had been hung over the entire district. I had been walking the entire day, so I was hungry and in search of *anything* to eat. Finally, in a stretch of plywood covered storefronts I came across a McDonalds. I went inside and got a milkshake. It wasn't until I sat down at a booth that I felt the stares. I was the only white person in the restaurant. My presence wouldn't have fazed anyone if this were the Caribbean, but folks here were glaring at me with unwelcome looks – perhaps even an air of surprise – as if to say, "what are *you* doing *here?*" I wasn't used to this. In the Caribbean, most folks would go out of their way to make a friendly connection and start a conversation.

Another sharp contrast was New York City. We were tied alongside the South Street Seaport Museum, just around the corner from Wall Street. Every lunch hour a row of crisp, clean, expensive suits lined up like perched black crows along the dock's balcony railing above the ship. Enviously peering down at the motley crew of dirty-tarred riggers and busy painters below, you could feel the yearning in them to dump it all and sail away to sea. They might have thought differently had they seen us a week earlier, clawing our way up the East coast against a raging Atlantic storm, barely making headway against the ravages of weather and tide.

After traversing the eastern seaboard we made landfall in Canada. In the Bras D'or Lakes of Nova Scotia a reporter from CBC Radio interviewed a group of the female trainees. Although, this reporter did not seem interested in the details of our travels and adventures at sea. He was digging for a story and was pushing the girls to reveal some fantastical romantic exchange on board that he had dreamt up. Much to the chagrin of the girls, he was making lewd remarks and suggestions. "*Surely* with all these young men and women on board there must be *something* going on?" When he actually used the words "hanky panky" I had finally had enough. I interjected and stated bluntly "There's a *watertight steel bulkhead door* separating the males and females." That shut him up, and the ladies of the forecastle seemed impressed by my direct delivery of the facts to him.

Our transit of the St. Lawrence River coincided with festivities in Ottawa marking Canada's 125th birthday. This included the entire crew paddling three enormous Voyageur canoes up the Rideau Canal. We were excited and keen. We had travelled so far on a traditionally built tall ship so it seemed fitting that we would paddle these historic craft. Strangely enough, they ended up being replicas made out of fiberglass and painted on the outside to look like they were clad in bark. How ironic that we had sailed so far on our well serving home of wood, only to have to represent Canada's marine heritage in these fake 'wanna-be-canoes'.

Kingston, Ontario was the final destination of this leg of the voyage. You would think being so far inland we would be safe from the effects of any major weather, but a strong spring storm had developed and we were forced to anchor opposite Kingston in the lee of Wolfe Island. With two enormous fisherman anchors splayed out before us, along with all of the associated heavy chain anchor rode and the ship's powerful diesel auxiliary spinning our prop at a good clip, we barely held our position in the bay. After the storm subsided we secured the vessel in Kingston, where a crew change took place. It was my time to fly home again, where I would once again work the summer with the S.A.L.T.S coastal program aboard the *Robertson II*.

CHAPTER SIX

THE CALAMITY KID

Monday, December 12, 2011 at 3:37pm

Jasper has just finished his first cycle of chemo and tomorrow he might be released from the hospital for a couple of days. We're not sure yet whether his next chemo cycle will happen before or after Christmas - it depends on his white blood cell counts. Either way, he is staying in Vancouver for the next few months and won't be able to travel home to Powell River. We found out today that we can stay at the Ronald McDonald House until at least January 10th. It is a good place for us to be over Christmas. We may still be looking for a place in Vancouver to stay in February, but we'll cross that bridge when we come to it. I think Jasper has almost enough stylish hats to wear a different one for everyday of the month now - so no need for folks to send him any more hats! Jasper is in good spirits. Sometime in the next week his hair is expected to fall out - so he figures it's a good time to dye it black.

Barb and I are both super tired but still keeping afloat. Onwards we go...

§

During the winter, the *Robertson II* would be laid-up until the next sailing season. I would work hard with the crew to do maintenance on the vessel: painting, varnishing, rigging repairs, etc. I'd be completely knackered by the end of the day, and filthy with wood dust, shavings, paint, glue and tar. Being so tired, it was always a struggle to make something to eat. It was usually toast or a baked potato. Thankfully, there were times that a crewmember would invite me home to a good home cooked meal with their family. Perhaps I'd even get a hot shower.

I was living aboard the *Robertson II* and acting as Shipskeeper. The position entailed tending to the ship's safekeeping at night; adjusting dock lines, securing items on deck from passing storms, and playing the role of a night watchman. More than once it involved kicking the drunken crowd out of the rigging when the local bar emptied out at two in the morning. Twice I was awoken by drunks who had found their way below deck and were traipsing through my cabin. Fortunately, I was not staying aboard that Christmas Eve, the year an escaped mental hospital patient decided to enter the vessel wielding a fire axe.

It was always an effort to stay warm on board. The tiny woodstove in the aft cabin needed constant attention by feeding it scraps of wood. I wasn't the only resident seeking out warm quarters. There was a compliment of several other inhabitants on the vessel. There were two large rats that I affectionately named *Ernie* and *Bert*. Thankfully their stay was quite short-lived. There was a raccoon that would transit the ship's decks every night. I could hear him rummaging around somewhere above my head as he scavenged in the dark. The ship also had an infestation of June bugs and cockroaches. Many a night I climbed into my sleeping bag, wearied and worn from a day of heavy work, to be greeted by the sensation of these critters scurrying around next to my skin. Nothing that couldn't be cured by a couple of good quick body rolls back and forth though. Then I would fall into a deep sleep, within sight of the warm glow of the woodstove and the crackle and pop of the fire inside it.

One evening, some trainees who had previously sailed aboard the ship were accompanying their friend, introduced to me as Barb, for a tour of the vessel. Needless to say, Barb's first impression of me when I stuck my head out of the companionway hatch, looking like the proverbial 'Wild man from Borneo' with my dirty face and long hair full of debris from a day's work, was that I must be some sort of young, delinquent, hard-case that S.A.L.T.S had taken under their wing in an act of compassion. She came across to me as a bit of a snob, and when they left I thought nothing more of Barb Hulsker.

In 1992 I was asked to join the crew of the *Pacific Swift* in Seville, Spain as the ship's Boatswain. Like many Christian non-profit groups, despite the portrayal that everything is rosy on the outside, often the staff are treated poorly within the organization. S.A.L.T.S was no exception, particularly with acts of favoritism and nepotism. If you didn't like how something was done - get out of the way, because you were expendable and there was a long line of eager replacements more than happy to take your place. When I was offered the role of Boatswain I knew that I was essentially filling the position of a crewmember that had voiced some dis-satisfactions. I felt a bit conflicted when they offered me the job, as the fellow who had turned it down was also a friend. But the chance to sail the ship home from Europe was an opportunity too great to pass up, and so I accepted. Although I've since discussed the situation with that friend, and he has told me not to worry about it, I can't help but feel that I might have stabbed him in the back by not turning down the job as a sign of support to him. I had also come to the conclusion that if I had chosen not to go, they would have just offered it to the next chum in line. Looking back now, if I had not gone, I wouldn't have met Barb once again...

When I journeyed to Spain to join the ship, I delivered a sack of mail for the crew on board. In this package of mail was a clipping from a local newspaper. It was a story about a young lady from Calgary, Alberta, who was travelling abroad. She seemed to be avoiding a catastrophe of major proportion everywhere she visited. I recognized the name and the included photo as Barb. Apparently she had left London's theater district just hours before a theater was bombed. In Amsterdam an El Al jumbo jet crashed into an apartment building where she had just been previously walking. While visiting Cairo she left for a daytrip to Scuba dive in the Red Sea, during which time Cairo experienced a devastating earthquake. Her penchant for avoiding these disasters started circulating back home through Barb's mother, who was kept on pins and needles for news of Barb's well being. It seemed that Barb had become a bit of a local celebrity in Alberta. A radio station would regularly telephone her mother for an update on the 'Calamity Kid' as they dubbed her.

Now, Barb was due to join the *Pacific Swift* in Spain.

Some warning bells should have signaled in my head to avoid this girl and her path of destruction at all costs. Instead I thought, "Cool... I think I know her," slung the mailbag over my shoulder, and went on my way to join the boat in Spain.

CHAPTER SEVEN

NUTMEG MILKSHAKES

Saturday, December 17, 2011 at 8:51am

Still quarantined in the room for at least the weekend. Blood counts are all very low. He's had a fever all night long. His eye infection is clearing up. It looks like we'll be in the hospital over Christmas, so we put a tree up in Jasper's room!

Thursday, December 22, 2011 at 8:25pm

We broke out of quarantine for a couple of hours and went to the Christmas lights display at Van Dusen Gardens. I'm giving Jasper a bottle of 'Old Spice' cologne for Christmas. Because, like their commercial states: "Anything is possible when your man smells like Old Spice!"

§

"Just so you know, you were not my first choice for this position." Well, that made me feel pretty small right off the mark, and it soured a relationship with the new Skipper. That is what he declared to me when I boarded the ship in Seville, Spain for the start of the voyage.

As the Boatswain aboard the trip, it was my job to maintain all the varnish and paint, tend to the upkeep of the rigging and sails, and stay on top of the regular maintenance and running of the auxiliary engine. As the ship was one hundred and eleven feet long overall, there was always something to do. There were thirty of us aboard, split into three 'watches' that rotated through a schedule of eating, sleeping, and sailing duties. Everyone would fall comfortably into this regular routine aboard the vessel. The vibrant busy life aboard the ship at sea proved to be an exciting little microcosm of its own. It was a terrific way to see the world. Sailing into the port of a country by way of a ship is an entirely different experience than arriving by airplane or automobile.

"Sail south until the butter melts" is the old adage of sailors looking to make an east-to-west Atlantic crossing, and we aimed to do just that. We were to sail from Spain to the Islands of Madeira, south to the Canaries and Africa's Cape Verde before crossing the Atlantic to the Caribbean. We would then transit the Panama Canal and do a tour of the South Pacific that included the Galapagos Islands, the Pitcairn Islands, the French Marquesas, Hawaii, and then home to British Columbia.

Whenever the ship was in port, the Boatswain had a lot of provisioning and repairs to do that couldn't happen while being at sea. When my duties were finished and I was able to get ashore, I aimed to maximize my time and experience in these new foreign destinations. Some of the trainees on board were complacent and ventured out no further than the local ice cream parlor. Others had designs similar to mine: to go find an adventure. Barb was one of the trainees that were keen to explore and experience what our destinations had to offer. We were like-minded in that way.

It all started with the two of us commiserating together over nutmeg milkshakes overlooking the Carenage of St. George's, Grenada. My workday was complete and I needed to get ashore for a break and a change of scenery. I climbed up on deck from below to find Barb crying in the arms of another female crewmember. She was upset having received a letter from a travel companion from her past. Apparently this fellow was expressing his wishes to join her on the boat. Barb had worked very hard to afford a berth on this voyage, and taking part in this trip was something she wanted to do on her own, especially without the baggage of a past relationship of any type. She was building up the situation in her head and it was upsetting her. How was she going to reply and what was she supposed to tell this guy? I told her it was simple. "Just tell him straight out: No!" She liked that uncomplicated solution. She looked like she needed cheering up, so I invited her then and there for a nutmeg milkshake. She wiped away some tears and smiled. Close by there was an open-air restaurant on the second floor of a building that had a great view of the harbor, and the best nutmeg milkshakes imaginable. Barb and I found we had much in common. It was easy to talk to each other. I was feeling downtrodden by the constant scrutiny of the Skipper, so I was happy to be able to share my plight with someone. We soon became good friends. We enjoyed each other's company and started spending a lot of time together hiking, snorkeling, and camping on excursions ashore. She would plan the adventures, and when I was done my work I would quickly throw some essentials into a backpack and we would head off to explore.

Our friendship flourished quickly into something more. Relationships aboard the ship were shunned – especially between a crewmember and a trainee (even though we were the same age) so we kept it hidden. Our friendship grew even stronger and we fell in love. We would secretly pass each other love letters. We each used an alias in case a letter was somehow intercepted onboard. I was *'Solo'* and she was *'Scarlet'*. We started making plans for a future together. I proposed to Barb in the French Marquesas on the island of Hiva Oa. It was so romantic, the stuff of fairy tales. It was a beautiful evening, and we ran through a field of grass with the sky pouring down warm rain from a passing squall. Seeking shelter from the rain, we stood under the eaves of an open lean-to shelter that had a thatched grass roof. We were just out of sight from a fellow trainee. He was inside playing his saxophone to a single candle illuminating the structure. I tucked a Frangipani into Barb's hair. It could not have been more perfect.

We kept the special news to ourselves for the next few days. We wanted to let our parents know before it became the public knowledge of everyone on board. We were anchored in Taiohae Bay off the island of Nuku Hiva when Barb and I decided to take advantage of an available telephone ashore to call our families. I sheepishly approached the Skipper to ask for permission to go ashore. He responded sternly "No. There's too much work here to be done." Okay. Would it be all right to use the Ham Radio on board? (Dad happened to be one of the amateur radio contacts that the ship regularly checked in with.) "No, wait until we check in tonight. Why do you need to use it right now?" We hesitantly explained that we were engaged and wanting to break the news to our parents. I was waiting for his gruff reply, but his stern face melted away into a great big smile – he was very happy for us. He ushered us off to use the island's telephone right away.

There were two telephones available ashore at the post office, and they were right beside each other. So it was, that Robin, a fellow trainee who was phoning home herself, overheard our news. She almost dropped her phone. We explained to her how we wanted to keep it a secret for a few days before telling everyone else aboard. Keeping this sweet bit of gossip to herself would prove to be hard for her, as back home she was an emerging television news reporter. It was a shock to everyone on the ship when we finally announced our engagement a few days later – and a huge relief to Robin. She had been going crazy trying to contain our secret. Our news was such a surprise to everyone. A lot of the crew hadn't realized we were even close friends, let alone in love.

The ship arrived in Hawaii. This was where a change of trainees would take place before the final voyage home to Victoria, British Columbia. Barb had completed her allotted time aboard so she took a flight home to Canada. I telephoned her to check in before we left Hawaii. At first, when she answered the call, she didn't know who it was. She hadn't recognized me because we had never spoken over the phone before. Our relationship was rowboats and remote beaches and treks through the jungle and nutmeg milkshakes. How odd that we had never spoken over a phone, or even gone out to dinner and a movie together.

I continued as Boatswain for the final offshore leg home to British Columbia. We were due to sail into Victoria where a planned celebration for the completion of the voyage would take place. I should have known better then to let the 'Calamity Kid' leave the ship. Sure enough, several hundred nautical miles north of Hawaii there was a loud BANG! The propeller shaft had sheared in two, causing the actual propeller to shift aft and wedge itself into the rudder. We were essentially without power, and without steerage. The evening sky was growing dark. Several of us dove down over the side to inspect the damage and clear away the wreckage. We managed to regain the steering, but there was no possibility of repairing the propeller shaft. Without an engine, we were at the mercy of the wind for the rest of the trip home.

The first week produced slow days with a lack of wind. We drifted fruitlessly under a hot sun. We then came into the trade winds that would carry us homeward. Soon after, the weather turned sour and the winds rose to incredible speeds. The wind began ripping sails faster than we could re-stitch them.

I remember being aloft stitching a sail from the end of the starboard yardarm, sixty feet above the deck. The boat was yawing severely side-to-side in the heavy seas. At each termination of the pendulum's swing there would be a mighty lurch. This would cause the yardarm and all of its associated gear to jolt violently in its slings, leaving me hanging on for my life. Then, as the mast and yard swung an arc across to the opposite horizon, I would quickly try to get a stitch or two more into the torn sail before the next jolt. I was working twenty feet out on the end of the starboard yard. The ship was rolling back and forth so far, that if I had fallen, I would have disappeared into the sea well off the opposite (port) side of the vessel.

Working aloft in these challenging conditions was exhausting. It was quite a chore to keep up with the constant necessary repairs to the ship in this weather. Then, we badly ripped the mainsail. We placed it on deck and all hands turned to stitching this fifty-foot long tear down the entire trailing edge of the sail. I set up a trainee with a sail needle and twine every four feet for the length of the ship, with every last needle from my Boatswain's stores. I was exhausted. I would take a short break in the aft cabin, cold and soaking wet on the inside of my foul weather gear. The unrelenting Skipper saw me and laid into me with a yell. "Aren't you in the least bit concerned we have a giant rip in the mainsail?" Stricken by this uncalled-for guilt trip he had laid upon me, I slunk back to work on deck in the rain. He went back to his warm cabin to study his charts.

We were weeks behind schedule and everyone's patience was wearing thin. I was perpetually tired and I missed Barb. The weather was not getting any better, and now we were running low on food stocks. We had plenty of lentils though, and the cooks started adding them copiously to every meal. God, to this day I don't want to eat another lentil.

Day after day we continued to rip sails and break gear. The ship was stuck in an uncomfortable cycle of pitching and rolling from ear to ear. The deck was awash with never-ending combers and a flushing wall of waves. Our forward progress was frustratingly slow. We just didn't get a break.

I remember standing with Mark, a tall brawny trainee, on the fore deck. The bow was being heaved skywards and plummeting downwards through an arc of thirty feet or more. Plumes of dark water were thrown sideways over our heads. The wind whistled through the rigging behind us and a dull lead colored sky lay stretched out before us.

Mark asked with a hint of nervousness in his voice, "Do you think we're going to make it?" The ship started its downward plunge, leaving us with a momentary weightless sensation.

"Yeah. We can't be more than ten days from Canada now." Big curls of water surged up around the bulwark railings as we bottomed out on our fall from the sky. The ship buried her nose into the froth.

"But do you think we're going to *make* it?" he asked. Again, the deck tilted and lifted skywards.

Geez - he was asking how much more the ship could take. "Eh? ...Oh. Yeah man, we'll make it. She's been through a lot worse than this. She's seen at least two cyclones before. Don't worry..."

I turned my collar up towards the cold pelting rain and sea spray. I hadn't considered the possibility that we mightn't survive this last leg home. Now the seed of doubt was planted in my mind too...

Yes, we would eventually make it. Three weeks behind schedule, we would sail into the Strait of Juan de Fuca where a tugboat was waiting on station to tow us the remaining fifty miles to Victoria and I would soon be reunited with Barb. We made it home, but *The Calamity Kid* had struck again.

CHAPTER EIGHT

YOGURT & COFFEE BEANS

Monday, January 2, 2012 at 6:15am
If Jasper's vitals are all good he will get discharged today. The second cycle of chemo has been much easier on him than the first. In the next couple of weeks he will be poked and prodded again: MRI, audiology, stem cell harvest, etc., and most likely the surgery to remove the tumor. We've got confirmation that between treatments we can stay at the Ronald McDonald House until at least April. Jasper likes the Ronald McDonald House.

Wednesday, January 4, 2012 at 9:58pm
Jasper's pretty tired at this point, as his blood counts are so low. He's still smiling though. Onwards we go...

Monday, January 9, 2012 at 10:47am

Vomiting, high temperatures, and low blood counts today. The break in-between chemo cycles has been cut short and Jasper is admitted again.

Monday, January 16, 2012 at 8:17pm

Jasper's almost over his infections and about to be released from the hospital, but he's now caught a cold and will be put in isolation for 11 days. He just doesn't seem to get a break. Tomorrow is his stem cell harvest.

Wednesday, January 18, 2012 at 10:05pm

This evening we got moved up to isolation on floor 3B. The room has the worst cot I've slept on here yet. My head is in a hole, my chest is flexed upwards, my bottom is in a crater and my feet are elevated higher than my head! Tomorrow will be a big day for Jasper: 1 - Possible stem cell harvest in the morning if his counts are high enough. He'll be hooked up to a loud humming machine for several hours while it collects stem cells from his bloodstream. Painless. 2 - If his counts are still too low to collect the stem cells he'll have another GFR - a kidney function test. 3 - At 3:00pm he's scheduled for an MRI. This is a pretty epic scan as it will show the effects chemo has had on the tumor and will determine the next course of action to heal Jasper (surgery, radiation, chemotherapy, etc.). Currently: He's caught a cold and is stuck in isolation for who knows how long. Barb and I are both tired. The three of us are in good spirits. Onwards we go...

§

Upon returning from the offshore voyage, I worked the following season for S.A.L.T.S in their coastal sailing program. Barb and I were living together in a very tiny apartment in Oak Bay in Victoria. We decided to buy a vehicle, and we found an old 1968 Land Rover that needed some love. It was... somewhat drive-able. I say it was a 68', but it was such a decrepit mish mash of parts from throughout the 60's that it more accurately could be called a nineteen-sixty-jalopy. It was rough, even by Land Rover standards. For one, the gas tank was filled from the inside of the vehicle. This released a constant nauseating reek of fumes with the high potential of explosion. There was no insulation or headliner adorning the interior. That made for a noisy ride. It was so loud that we were forced to shout at each other to have a conversation. We grew used to this, and eventually gave up conversing in the truck altogether. Actually, there was no interior fitted at all save for a bench seat across the front of the cab. When Dad first saw this truck he thought it was completely unsafe and un-roadworthy. His plea of concern fell on deaf ears though, as I was completely in love with the beast. In a true East Indian television drama fashion, he told me that if I chose to drive this vehicle I was "out of the family!" He then stomped away in his flip-flop sandals to the seclusion of his Ham Radio shack, slamming the door behind him.

Barb and I took the *'Sugarbear'* on a camping trip in Washington State. As we pulled into a campsite a fellow camper ran up to us eagerly exclaiming "I can fix that for you!" I looked at him dumbfounded – fix what? "Well, you're only running on three cylinders." I hadn't even noticed. Well, truthfully I had noticed the long lines of cars stuck behind us in our slow wake. No wonder the truck had seemed so gutless. It needed no end of repairs. While I was at sea on the boat, Barb would be home rebuilding the truck's clutch master cylinder on the living room floor, parts and tools splayed everywhere. When I returned home there would be no evidence of her heavy mechanic wrenching whatsoever.

Although we were engaged and had a date to be married that autumn, there was chatter among the Christian S.A.L.T.S staff that we shouldn't be living together. It was also at this time that the Skipper had taken a shine to some new up and comer, so I was encouraged to move on (i.e. let go). This was unfortunate, as they were about to embark on the building of a new ship, which of course was my dream job. However, being away from Barb for most of the summer on the sailing trips wasn't ideal anyways, and the S.A.L.T.S wage was pretty meager. I reluctantly moved on.

By now I had amassed a substantial amount of 'sea time' and I considered further training to acquire a license and pursue a career at sea. The problem was that every licensed position required stereoscopic vision. This was the first time in my life that my vision had prevented me from pursuing a particular path. Not one to give up easily, I met with a top official Coast Guard Examiner to contest my case, but to no avail - I would need both eyes to hold any type of Mariner's ticket.

As our wedding day grew closer, four different fellows appeared unexpectedly out of the woodwork to announce their love for Barb. They pleaded for her to consider their case before marrying me. Oh brother! Two were old boyfriends who were yearning to reestablish a relationship. The other two had been casual friends of hers, and now they were breaching the limits of that past friendship and claiming that they had loved her since they had first laid eyes upon her. She felt a bit betrayed by these guys. They had been a friend and a co-worker - in a non-romantic way. Here they were, out of the blue, telling her they'd always been madly in love with her. They asked her to give up on me, and to run away with them to some fantasy world. I found it super annoying. Of course Barb assured me that I had nothing to worry about. But gee-whiz guys, *really*? It was so evident that we were in love and going to be married. Couldn't they have simply taken the high road and wished us well?

Barb and I were married on a glorious day in October of 1993 in my parent's garden in Qualicum Beach. It was a 'pot-luck' affair and folks brought everything from dishes of butter-chicken to sides of smoked salmon. It was a beautiful celebration. We drove away together in a borrowed 1960's VW camper van to Galiano Island for our honeymoon.

Back in Victoria, I found a job driving a delivery truck for a supply chain. I breezed through the interview process with flying colors, and then I was taken through the back door into the warehouse to meet the staff. "Would you like a coffee, Stephen?"

"No, thanks. I don't drink the stuff. I don't really like coffee." Silence. It was then it dawned on me that this was a warehouse filled to the rafters with coffee beans. Oops. I was to deliver coffee beans to the greater Victoria area. Barb and I would laugh how I was permitted to bring home free bags of coffee, even though neither of us drank it.

Barb had found a job too. She worked as a manager for a frozen yogurt kiosk in the mall. I would tease her that she was using her Biology degree to study bacteria cultures. She promptly quit the job when the owners refused her request to have the day of our wedding off from work.

Barb and I hatched a plan to travel two-up by motorcycle throughout Mexico. You would think I had learned something from my previous motorcycle accident in the Dominican Republic, but the temptation of travelling on two wheels into warmer climates was strong. This time, I took a motorcycle training skills course and acquired my license. Unlike in the Caribbean, this time I would be wearing a helmet too.

We loaded up a Kawasaki KLR650 and pointed it southwards. Space was limited with two of us riding on one small bike. We would each get a single side case for our clothes and toiletries, and a top case would house our food and camp stove. Somewhere in the jumble we strapped our sleeping mats, sleeping bags, a tent, and a telescopic fishing rod too. We fought a lot on that trip. We really should have bought a separate motorcycle for Barb to ride. We rode down the west coast in late fall, greeted everywhere we went by wind and rain. At least there were no major accidents to report. The closest thing we could call crashing was upon reaching Cabo San Lucas. Forced to make a choice of going left or right at a fork in the road, and myself being unprepared to make said choice, I kept us going on a course straight ahead. Despite Barb's protests from behind me to "Go left! No! Right! Where... No!" we crawled forward at a low speed into some soft deep sand that brought us to a full stop. Then the bike, its burden of gear, and the two of us all canted over in slow motion. It softly plopped itself down into the sand with its wheels in the air, us laughing the entire way as we were pulled down with it. Always make a grand entrance when given the opportunity.

We made the decision to cut the trip shorter than we had originally planned and ride home again, but not before journeying to the mainland of Mexico via a ferry from La Paz to Topolobampo. We arrived early to board the ferry, confident that we would have a spot as we were on a motorcycle. The boarding procedure took all day. The staff started by loading all of the semi-trailer trucks onto the vessel in reverse. Many of these trucks had to be backed onto the ferry and then directed up the incline of an internal ramp to the second deck. It was hot in the parking lot and there was no shelter from the sun. By late afternoon none of the passenger vehicles had been boarded yet, and the staff looked like they were closing the gates and preparing to depart. I started the bike and made for the gate. We were stopped, some garbled Spanish was shouted back and forth on the attendant's radio, and we were directed up the ramp. Other than the semi-trailer trucks, we were the only ones to be let on the ferry. Good thing too, as I don't think I could have managed another day standing idle in the blistering sun like that. Little did I know what frigid temperatures I would soon have to endure when we made the trip north past Mount Shasta in a November snowstorm.

Upon our return home to Victoria, Barb volunteered for the local Marine Mammal Research Group. A scientist who seemed to subsist on Coca-Cola and toast ran the organization. Barb would enter recorded sightings of dolphins or whales into a database for him. Occasionally she would help perform a necropsy on a porpoise or some other sad dead mammal that had washed ashore on the tide. It was through this job that she caught wind of a position at a whale watching company.

Seacoast Expeditions was the first whale-watching outfit to work out of Victoria's Inner harbor. They had three high-speed rigid hulled inflatables that would each carry twelve passengers, a pilot to operate the vessel, and a qualified naturalist. Not to be confused with naturist, the naturalist (fully clothed) was a wildlife expert that would inform the passengers about what they were viewing. Trips were three hours long and tailored around viewing the resident killer whale population. Barb started as a naturalist with Seacoast and then trained as a pilot for the vessels. Later on she would take on the role of general manager.

Meanwhile, although I didn't mind driving the giant Grumman delivery van, I grew tired of coming home at the end of the day smelling of cardboard and coffee beans. I accepted a position with Seacoast as a 'Spotter'. It was my job to find the whales and direct the boats to them. I would carry massive four-feet long high-powered binoculars and a large wooden tripod to the top of Mount Douglas each morning. From here I would scan the horizon for the telltale spouting breaths of whales, then radio my findings to the boats. These were very powerful binoculars. From Mount Douglas, I could pick out individual people on the waterfront of San Juan Island – more than ten kilometers away.

With my background in boats, it was fitting that I too should become a pilot with the company. These were the early days of watching whales in the area. Our passengers were keen, adventuresome folks who were genuinely interested and amazed at anything you showed them. We saw some amazing sights. We witnessed whales mating, or tearing a seal apart, or using our boat as a tool to trap a salmon against. We saw young killer whale calves playing in beds of bull kelp while squeaking out sounds of pleasure as they rolled over in the fronds. Every trip of every day was met with the anticipation of a different spectacle.

Some folks interpreted their experience with the whales quite differently than others. There was a group that regularly chartered one of our boats for an entire afternoon every year. We nicknamed them *'The Crystal Draggers'*. The group embraced a belief that they shared some type of spiritual connection with the whales. They would light smelly incense and sing and hum and drag crystals behind the boat. I imagine they're the type that owns a gaudy velvet painting depicting a killer whale breaching in front of a waterfall under a full moon.

I was more inclined to think we were watching the ocean's equivalent of a herd of cows. But then every once in a while I would be shown something incredible that I couldn't explain, and it would remind me that these creatures may indeed be some higher level sentients.

One close encounter I will remember for the rest of my days. Sometimes the whales would pass right underneath the boat. There was one instance that I found haunting. I had a thirty-foot long killer whale bull turn on to his side and look me directly in the eye as he passed. It was a soul-piercing stare that went right into me. His look almost seemed to say, "I am going to remember you." Then he surfaced and exhaled so close that I breathed his breath. We had both looked deep inside each other, and we had shared the same life-giving breath. There was a connection made that day. It left me with the feeling that I had to be accountable for my actions when I was out on the water around the whales.

We observed lots of other wildlife on our expeditions too. Humpback and Grey whales would breach right beside us. We would watch harbor seals basking in the sunshine. Pacific White-sided Dolphins would occasionally make an appearance, travelling in groups of well over a hundred and entertaining us with their acrobatics. Groups of Dall's Porpoises would ride the bow wave of the boat. We would visit the island group called Race Rocks where I would nose the bow of the boat directly beneath the perch of a Stellar sea lion that was the size of a VW Beetle. There were multitudes of birds in the area: eagles, cormorants, tufted puffins, grebes, shearwaters, petrels, pelicans, herons, ducks, oystercatchers, gulls, loons, and vultures. The naturalists that worked on board with me were so knowledgeable. Their stories and interpretations of our surroundings could be mesmerizing. They could make a simple seagull sound exciting.

The naturalists took their job very seriously. Occasionally I would attempt to interject some lightness into their fact-filled wildlife documentary. "Oh! And look at that folks: a flamingo! What a rare sighting." This mocking would result in a reprimanding sharp elbow to my ribs from Heather or Tian - "Stephen!" For a while I tried to start a ridiculous rumor amongst them that a saltwater crocodile had been spotted off the Victoria waterfront – but I don't think any of them were buying it. They were suspicious of any claims I made to rare creature sightings from that day forward.

One of my favorite memories was an evening trip, the sky above Haro Strait a glowing solid band of orange, the water glassy calm, and me surrounded on all sides as far as I could see by a 'super-pod' of killer whales. This was a rare occurrence when all the resident pods would combine into one enormous gathering. We had a hundred killer whales all to ourselves with not another boat in sight.

I stayed with Seacoast for five years. Barb was there for six. We left when the original owner sold the company. We got out just in time, as now the industry is a bit of a circus with an inordinate number of vessels all competing to see a smaller population of whales. Nowadays whale watching appears more akin to a bus tour that merely wants to put a bum in a seat for cash.

Barb and I weren't finished with the sea though. We started looking into purchasing a small boat of our own. On one of her visits from Alberta, Barb's mother brought us a 'gift'. It was a wrecked ten-foot-long, dilapidated old English sailing dinghy she had found behind a barn. I set about restoring it with the plan that Barb and I could enjoy some sailing together. I spent my spare time steam bending new oak frames into it and stripping back layers of old paint. The boat still had its original 'Gunter' rig, and I made repairs to the spars and hung them from the ceiling in our small apartment, where we applied coat upon coat of varnish to them. We had a small launch party in Oak Bay where we christened the boat *'Robin'*. We named it after our shipmate friend - the same Robin we sailed with on the *Pacific Swift* who was the first to hear of our engagement. Sadly, shortly after Robin had returned home from her travels, she died in a plane crash. We felt this was a good way to honor her memory.

It was quite comical to watch us sail this boat in Oak Bay. Barb comes from a background of competitive small boat racing. Thus she was always trying to get the maximum performance from *Robin*, telling me to shift my weight forward or to move my butt to the opposite side of the boat (in not such polite terms). I was more from the camp that just wanted to lie on my back and watch the mast moving against the passing clouds. Clearly we were not on the same page in this boat. Barb would put the dinghy through its paces, often sailing it on its ear. It was fantastic fun. We received many concerned glances from passing boats, scrutinizing our sanity of being so far out from shore in such a tiny open boat. This would prove to be the only boat in our marriage that we would fight aboard. One time Barb had actually considered jumping overboard and leaving me to my devices. We began to think about a bigger sailboat: one that we could live aboard.

This plan was abruptly put on hold, when in 1994, Barb detected a lump on her neck. A doctor told her that it was likely just a swollen lymph node and that it would soon disappear. It didn't go away, so she got a second doctor to look at it and take a biopsy. She was diagnosed with thyroid cancer. A surgery was scheduled and they completely removed her thyroid leaving her with a scar across her neck. She kidded that she had been in a sword fight with an immortal Scottish Highlander that had tried to cut her head off. During her recovery I would climb into her hospital bed to read books to her. Would she survive this? It had been a long time since I had last had any concerns about cancer in my family. I had never dreamed that Barb would get the disease. I always thought that if it showed itself again it would be in me.

Following surgery Barb had to have radioisotope therapy. This involved flushing her system with a radioactive form of iodine to remove any traces of thyroid tissue. She was placed in isolation for four days under the restriction of no visitors. I felt so alone and scared for her. I couldn't visit her, so I had to get creative in order to see her. Outside the hospital, I would pull myself up a low brick wall to the window ledge of her room. I could support myself on my elbows for about a minute before I would have to fall back down to the grass below, have a short rest, and scale the wall again to peer through the glass. Then repeat. The window didn't open, but at least we could see each other. I was so worried about the chance that I might lose her to cancer if this treatment didn't go as planned.

These were tough times. Dad also had a brush with danger and was diagnosed with colon cancer. Fortunately they caught it early and it was small, so they were able to resect his colon. Dad was back to his usual self in short order. It was found that he did have rather high blood pressure though. Many men of East Indian descent can be prone to high blood pressure. For the future he would have to keep a close eye on it and take medication to keep it in check. Although he was given a status of remission, some of the medications he was prescribed would later take a toll on his circulation system.

When Barb came home from isolation she was mildly radioactive for two weeks. Because of my cancer history, we were not allowed to be within two meters of each other for this period. That was not going to be an easy feat in our tiny apartment. We were not permitted to touch similar surfaces either; things like cutlery or dishes or chairs.

After receiving radioisotope therapy, it is highly recommended to wait a full year before having a child. We were hoping to have a baby, but this decided for us. We would have to wait.

One year later they did a test to see if any thyroid tissue had remained. Indeed, sadly it did show up in the tests. So once again Barb had to have the radioactive therapy and be placed in isolation. Hopefully this would rid her of any remaining thyroid tissue. It was quite taxing on us both to go through this routine again of having treatment and then waiting a full year to see the results. We would have to be patient for yet another full year before even considering having a baby.

Finally, the following year she was given the all clear. We could now pursue our dream of making a family. We were concerned that a baby might inherit my retinoblastoma cancer gene, so we met with a geneticist at

Victoria General Hospital. I remember him as being quite condescending toward us, to the point of speaking like we were kindergarten students. There was a fifty-fifty chance that the gene would be passed along and an eighty percent chance the child could then get cancer if he did indeed inherit the gene. It equaled a forty percent chance overall. Not entirely the best odds, but we were hopeful and wanted so badly to have a family. Also, seeing as how I had survived my cancer, we didn't view it as incurable if that was the outcome.

Three months into her pregnancy Barb had a miscarriage. This was disheartening to say the least, and we were left wondering if we could ever have a baby. But Barb soon became pregnant again.

About four months into the pregnancy the baby made its first attempt at communication with us. It was a frigid week in December. We had borrowed the schooner *'Dana Erin'* from a friend for a cruise. A week of winter sailing on the cold coast of British Columbia for fun would seem a legitimate reason for anyone to question our sanity. We were hoping to enjoy some off-season sailing, enticed by the prospect of empty anchorages void of other boats. And we were correct: there was no one else out here, because no one in their right mind would contemplate a cruise for pleasure at this time of year. Winter on the coast brings strong weather: high winds, relentless rain, and a biting chill that penetrates right through all the layers you've wrapped your body in. The looming Solstice equates to minimal hours of usable daylight, and the broad range of

December's tides produces strong moving currents. It's no wonder the anchorages are empty.

Dana Erin was an engineless wooden boat, only twenty feet in length. If you weren't sailing her, you could propel her by sweeping a 'yuloh' (a long oar) off the stern. The yuloh on board *Dana Erin* seemed a little short to me, so I borrowed one from the junk-rigged *'China Cloud'*, somehow convincing myself that this longer version would make us faster by leaps and bounds. I soon learned that sculling a boat against the tidal races of Boundary Pass is a slow endeavor; no matter what size oar you stick out the back. The old adage applies: it's not the size of oar, but how you use it.

The boat was flush-decked, meaning that she had no cabin projecting above her deck, and as such she only had four feet of vertical height to her interior. This made her quite 'cozy' below decks, with room for one person to sit cross-legged in front of a small woodstove. This was possibly the smallest iron woodstove ever manufactured. Its firebox was capable of burning the equivalent of maybe a dozen wooden Popsicle sticks at a time. This was our source of heat. As a result of my six-foot tall frame, sitting in front of the fire in the hopes to get warm meant the top of my head would project outside, exposed to the elements. Just forward of the coveted spot of the woodstove were the miniscule sleeping quarters, where lying on your back in the cold you could witness your breath reflecting off the underside of the deck, a mere four inches from the end of your nose. The coffin-like space was so tight that any conjugal relations were out of the question. Getting into this bunk necessitated a commitment to stay there for the long term. With all the effort required, it was not something you wanted to repeat often. From the boat's cockpit, I'd perform a Limbo dance maneuver to fold myself down the hatch. Once below, I would shimmy into my cold sleeping bag. To access the bunk would then require a backwards, prostrate, feet-first entry that resembled a fat polyester caterpillar waddling in reverse.

We were anchored for the night in Bedwell Harbor, Pender Island. The moon was full, the winter sky radiant with stars, and the wind light. Barb and I had just settled into our sleeping bags for the night. I was just starting to feel some semblance of warmth when Barb exclaimed, "The wind must have come up - our anchor is dragging."

"What? How do you figure that?"

"I heard the anchor chain through the hull," she stated.

Not being one to passively go back to sleep after such an announcement (especially since it was a borrowed boat), I went through the tedious exercise of ejecting myself from the interior of the vessel. Several minutes later, I stood in the cockpit facing the piercing cold night in nothing more than my underwear, and surveyed the situation. There was no wind or tide to speak of in the slightest. We were not dragging the boat's hook. Back to bed...

The fat caterpillar uttered a few choice words under his breath as he wiggled his way forward to regain his cocoon.

"Did you feel that? I'm sure we're dragging our anchor. I can feel the chain moving across the seabed below us."

Once again I endured the long pilgrimage to gain the deck. My investigations turned up no source. Back to bed... Limbo. Scrunch. Shimmy. Bangs forehead. (Expletive). Wiggle.

Shivering with cold, I crawled back into position beside Barb. There certainly wasn't any reason for this little boat to move from its well-placed hook.

It wasn't long before she announced, "There it is again! Did you feel *that*?"

I was becoming suspicious of her. "I'm so cold that I don't feel anything, Barb. There's no possible way we can be dragging our anchor. It's flat calm."

"Wait a second... There! Yes... I think... I think that must be the baby's first kicks!"

"What?" I went to sit up and bumped my head again.

"Here, feel this." She reached across and placed my hand on her belly. "Wait for it... There! Feel that?"

"Wow! No-way!" I exclaimed, unbelievably thrilled. "It's kicking! I can feel it in there. It seems to kick whenever we talk!"

And so it was that we happily determined the source of rumbling: not the anchor dragging, but the baby's first movements. It seemed fitting that this baby would already have close ties to boats and the sea. The boat's woodstove crackled away, and we both snuggled into our cocoons for a deep winter sleep, excited with the anticipation of the future birth of our own little butterfly.

On June 12, 1998 Barb gave birth to a beautiful baby boy at the Victoria General Hospital. We were completely ecstatic with joy.

CHAPTER NINE

JASPER SOLO

We had waited so long to have him. Now here he was – so beautiful, and healthy, and so... loud! The nurses at the Victoria General Hospital told me they had never heard such a loud baby before. When I spoke he would turn his head toward me. I think he recognized my voice because I read books to him in utero.

We named him Jasper Solo Mohan. 'Jasper' as I had lots of fond memories spent in Jasper National Park during my childhood. 'Solo' was a combination of my love letter alias and the character of Han Solo from the Star Wars films. It has connections to sailing as well. I really wanted him to have a unique name, and Solo conjures up connotations of being an individual in a sea of others. I joke often that we named him Solo because Barb said no to 'Vader'. After his birth we travelled to Jasper National Park and baptized him ourselves below the Athabasca Falls, just the three of us – a family, before God.

We had recently bought the sailboat we had been dreaming of and we lived aboard her in Oak Bay. *'Gamester'* was a thirty-two foot long English sloop built in 1939. She was finished out down below like an old English pub. High backed leather settees and the rich dark glow of mahogany abounded in the interior. Jasper had a bunk with extendable high sides to keep him safe when we had our hands full sailing the boat. We used to bathe him in the boat's dish bin. On sunny days outside, the cockpit was a giant safe playpen for him. It was a cozy home, just the right size for the three of us. We had lots of fun times sailing up and down the B.C. coast in this boat. We sailed her to the Port Townsend Wooden Boat Festival in Washington State. This was the largest gathering of wooden boats on the west coast. I had been to this festival a number of times as a spectator and always yearned to have a boat of my own present. I was proud to show our home to the festival attendees. It felt quite special to be a part of it all. We were somewhat of an anomaly, being a family that actually lived aboard.

Of course we had been dutifully diligent and on guard for any irregularities in Jasper's eyes. When Jasper was five months old we were dealt the blow that there might be tiny tumors growing in both eyes. God, please no. We immediately rushed off to the B.C. Children's Hospital in Vancouver, where the bad news was then confirmed.

What followed was laser and cryotherapy treatment to both of his eyes – every three weeks. This was gradually spread out to every three months until he was two years old. We got to know the routine at the hospital all too well. We were constantly back and forth on the ferry between Victoria and Vancouver. It was so hard and tiring on Barb and I. Sometimes we would stay in Vancouver at the Ronald McDonald House. The Ronald McDonald House provided us with a 'home away from home'. It's a charity set up for folks who have a child in treatment and need somewhere to stay. Most of the time we just wanted to get home again as soon as possible, so we'd make a sprint for the ferry in an attempt to get back to our own 'normal' lives.

 The treatments were exhausting. First thing in the morning we would check in to day surgery at the Children's Hospital. Day surgery was a busy place with lots of kids coming and going for all sorts of procedures. Jasper would be prepped in a loose yellow hospital gown and then administered multiple eye drops. Eye drops are not a fun experience for a toddler. He would then get a pre-surgery visit from the ocular tumor specialist and the anesthetist. We would wait for hours before his surgery time came up. He would play in the toy area, or climb into our laps so we could read to him. Soon the eye drops would take affect and he would become irritated, as he could no longer see clearly. He was usually hungry by now too, as he had been fasting for the surgery. The nurses in their operating garb would come fetch him when it was his turn. Barb would be permitted to walk into the operating theater with him. She would have to wear the hospital gown, hairnet, mask and slippers for this. I would make a wavering attempt at a brave goodbye to Jasper before he would disappear behind the doors into surgery.

He would be in there for at least an hour, and then his hospital bed was wheeled out to the recovery room. We would meet him there. He would still be asleep. He would spend up to an hour in recovery. When he awoke, his eyes would be a bit bloodshot. His voice would be scratchy from the anesthesia, so we would bring him popsicles. He was allowed as many popsicles as he wished. After he was feeling in better spirits, his bed would be wheeled back to the day surgery ward. Once the nurses were convinced he was fit enough to be released we would wrap him in blankets and carry him to our vehicle for the drive home. It was a full day affair. Eventually we fell into a routine where Barb would take him to these treatments, and I would take him to his chemotherapy sessions.

Chemotherapy started when he was eight months old. Being a new parent has enough challenges of it's own without throwing chemotherapy into the equation. By this point Jasper had a V.A.D. (venous access device) surgically implanted just below his collarbone. The V.A.D. would provide an access point for administering chemo and taking blood. Chemo for a baby is a horrible experience. He would throw up. The first time he vomited he had a puzzled look about it, as if to say, "what *is* that?" Then there were the diapers. 'Chemo diapers' full of toxic, burning chemicals were quite an unpleasant ordeal. I had to wear a full gown suit and gloves to change a diaper. It had to be done right away or it would burn his skin. And then the diaper would be disposed of as hazardous material. If I timed it right, his chemo would be administered right before his daily nap, giving us both an hour of rest. Each session would take half of a day. At least we were in Victoria at the general hospital for this treatment and we could readily go straight home afterwards. He had nine rounds of chemo up until he reached fourteen months old. Nine rounds is a lot of chemotherapy for anybody, let alone a baby. There was a big debate within the Tumor Board about this, as usually a patient is only prescribed six rounds.

 The treatments were effective against the tumors. We were so relieved. When Jasper reached three years old we were down to a check up with an Oncologist at B.C. Children's Hospital once a year. He would see the same Oncologist, Dr. Caron Strahlendorf, each time. Our visits with her got to be similar to visiting a family relative. It was a special relationship. Dr. Caron and Jasper would chat about all the events and experiences in Jasper's life the previous year. They would exchange book titles and discuss events at Jasper's school. She would give him a thorough check-up and then tell him he was doing "*absolutely* marvelous." He would be all smiles, and we'd head home.

 Barb and I made the decision not to have any more children. What if we had another child and they inherited the gene and became sick too? Did we have the strength to do this again? Thankfully, Jasper was too young to recall any of his experiences. That might not be the case if we had to relive it all again with a sibling and drag Jasper along through the ordeal. I was blissfully ignorant of my own treatment during my childhood. Because I was a baby when I had my cancer I have no recollection of the treatment. I could just go about being a kid, instead of being traumatized by hospitals and all the scary procedures that happen in them. We felt Jasper deserved that same bliss.

Jasper was an absolutely amazing child. For starters, he was very cute. People meeting him for the first time would remark on how beautiful his eyes were. If they only knew the story behind those eyes. And Jasper was smart - very smart. Off-the-charts smart.

He loved to read, and he started early at it. We never had a television in our home for his entire childhood, but we did buy him a Nintendo Gameboy - a hand held video game console. He played a game on it that had Lego 'mini-fig' people that spoke to each other with silent cartoon bubbles hanging over their heads. We quickly tired of reading these speech bubbles for him at each turn of the game, so we told him straight out, "If you want to play that game you will have to learn to read it yourself." Two or three days later he was reading it all on his own. He was *four*. How ironic that a video game taught a child to read. After that, his hunger for books was voracious. We couldn't feed him books fast enough. He would drop words he had read in his books into conversations with us – words he had read and understood the meaning of, but he hadn't ever heard pronounced yet. "It is just *chaw-us* outside, Mama" (chaos). His reading sprouted all manner of questions that he directed toward us, such as "Papa, what does it look like from the *inside* of a molecule looking *out*?"

Jasper would read to distraction. We once watched him walk out of the library with a new book held up to the end of his nose. He proceeded to open the door of someone else's car, get into the front passenger seat, and shut the door behind him as he continued reading. A minute later he noticed his mistake, but only because his nose had detected that this other car smelled badly.

When he entered the school system we had him tested for giftedness. He was off the charts. In fact, he was in the 99.9 percentile in every subject they tested him on. That meant out of every 1000 people there was only one person who would test as high as him. And that was in the normal population. It was then found that he ranked in the 96th percentile of the gifted population – meaning that only four in 1000 gifted people were testing as high or higher than him. His IQ was determined to be 145. To put that into perspective, only about five percent of the population scores above an IQ of 125. In short, he was a genius. He skipped ahead a grade level in school immediately, and we were constantly working with teachers to keep his hunger for knowledge satisfied as he progressed through the system.

Jasper was also very accepting. Upon meeting someone new, he would often proceed to climb up onto his or her lap and talk their ear off. This was a shock to a lot of people who weren't expecting it. Jasper could hold his own in a conversation with any adult. I had made a point to never speak to him in a condescending manner. I was so fortunate to be a stay-at-home dad with him. We did *everything* together. He had an incredible imagination and we would get up to all sorts of fun adventures. He could be completely independent too. He would walk down an entire stretch of beach before plopping himself down to play in the sand, oblivious to how far away I was.

Despite being played the cancer card early in his infant years, Jasper had a terrific childhood. He had lots of friends and his family loved him very much. He cherished the idea of an extended family with a network of relatives. Every summer he would spend some time with Grandma and Grandpa in Qualicum Beach. They would play on the beach, or go horseback riding, or do some serious baking together in the kitchen. Then he would travel to Calgary to visit his Oma and Opa, and his Aunt and Uncle. They would take him to the Calgary Stampede, or enroll him in the sailing school on Lake Chestermere, or go for a ride in their sports car.

Jasper made quite a lasting impression on folks. People would tell us that they thought he was the kind of person who could really make a difference in this world. On several occasions, couples would confide in us that it was meeting Jasper that had convinced them to have children of their own.

CHAPTER TEN

CARLOTTA

Thursday, January 19, 2012 at 9:54pm

Good news! This afternoon's MRI scan has shown the best possible outcome. The tumor has shrunk considerably and most of it is dead tissue. We are all greatly relieved. So surgery and radiation may not be necessary. Chemo will commence again next week with another possible time to collect stem cells again as we were unable to get them this time. Still looking at several months of chemotherapy ahead.

§

In 2003, we made a move to the city of Powell River, on the Sunshine Coast of B.C. Barb had gone back to school for an MBA degree and then found a respectable job as the city's Human Resources Manager. I balanced the role of a stay-at-home father with working part-time as a mechanic at Suncoast Cycles, the local bicycle shop. Although Powell River is only 175km north of Vancouver, to reach it you must take two consecutive ferries that run on limited schedules. It takes approximately five hours of travel time, *if* you time it correctly. If you don't time it right, or the weather is bad, or traffic is heavy, or the stars don't align, well... let's just say that I once flew from Vancouver to London in less time than the trip from Vancouver to Powell River.

Following the year of our move, Mom fell ill again. Her breast cancer came back, strangely enough appearing in the chest tissue of the breast that had previously been removed. It was frustrating for her, as she had been keeping really good care of herself. She was working for a fitness studio that promoted healthy lifestyles for seniors. She paddled with the local dragon boat team too. She felt cheated by becoming ill despite her healthy lifestyle. She started chemotherapy again, but the drugs were taking their toll on her, so she put her foot down and refused to take any more. Of course, the entire family was concerned about her rash choice of action. Barb and I respected her decision, but wondered if she had considered that maybe she shouldn't give up just yet, as she had a beautiful grandson to spend time with and watch grow up. She continued with radiation alone and began taking tamoxifen as a preventative measure. Thankfully, she again went into remission.

We had outgrown our boat *Gamester* and put it up for sale. We had a dream to own a larger boat to live aboard and travel on. I had my sights on owning a Bristol Channel pilot cutter. These were capable, seaworthy, working craft that many regarded as the penultimate of sailing vessels. They were built to transport a pilot out to an incoming ship off the rugged west coast of England in the days of gaff sail. They were stoutly built, as they had to operate in all seasons and all weather. They were fast boats too, as the pilots competed amongst each other to be the first to claim an incoming ship. Although at one point these boats numbered in the hundreds, there were now only a handful of them left – seventeen in fact, and all of them over the ripe old age of one hundred. It just so happened that one of these pilot cutters, *'Carlotta'*, was located in Gorge Harbor, Cortes Island, not far from us. Barb and I went to visit the boat, and although she looked more than a little rough around the edges, I instantly fell in love. Few boats can claim to be fast, beautiful *and* seaworthy. *Carlotta* checked each of these boxes for me. *Carlotta* had a reputation for winning races against vessels much bigger than her. She was capable of taking long ocean passages in stride, and being so stoutly built she could do this while giving her crew a sense of comfort, safety, and protection. Barb failed to see the appeal of such a vessel in its current state but saw that I was keen, so she ran with it. The current owner had sailed her for the past thirty-five years and wasn't ready to part with her quite yet, but we were subsequently invited to sail aboard a couple of times in the next few years.

One of these invitations was to help sail the boat at the Victoria Classic Boat Show. Barb and I joined the boat for the show's Sunday afternoon sail past. When we arrived

I offered to tidy up the lines on deck, which looked like they could use a bit of sorting and organizing. But Peter, the owner, took a more carefree attitude and told me not to worry about it. "Coiling lines is such a Sisyphean task, Stephen." Perhaps I was being too focused on keeping things in 'ship shape and Bristol fashion' from my days aboard the tall ships. Besides, it was a lazy autumn afternoon with barely a breeze in the air. What's the worst that could happen?

The sail past would involve a parade of classic wooden vessels each taking a turn at saluting a designated committee boat positioned at the entrance to Victoria harbor. This boat would have the Commodore and a group of dignitaries aboard. Also, the committee vessel was kind enough to hold onto our push boat for us so we could return safely under power into the busy harbor later in the day. *Carlotta* was an engineless vessel and relied on that push boat as a means of propulsion when necessary.

Next, there was to be an informal race for the sailboats. The race began in light airs with the competitors drifting lazily about. Unexpectedly, within an hour, a brisk wind had sprung up and escalated to the height of a full-blown gale. With the winds approaching forty knots we still carried full sail. We were going like a train. The sea was turbulently streaming past the hull and the odd cheeky wave of spray was reaching the crew. While the boat itself was built to take this sudden onslaught, some of the crew were not; we had a retired seagoing pilot and a maritime lawyer aboard as guests. Coincidentally, the lawyer's name was David Jones - sharing the same moniker from the infamous idiom *'Davey Jones' Locker'*, a euphemism for drowned sailors and their shipwrecks consigned to the bottom of the sea. Was his presence foreshadowing future events of the day? These guests' lazy afternoon drift while munching on tuna sandwiches was over. They both looked genuinely scared. Another lady aboard had brought her two children, who each suffered from Attention Deficit Disorder. They were confined down below, heavily drugged and sleeping. Un-stowed anchors and the odd heavy bar of lead ballast began crashing back and forth across the deck on each tack. I scampered about the decks securing items as best I could. A wooden fairlead mounted firmly into the deck could no longer bear the strain of the headsail sheets passing through it. It popped out and went spinning into the sea. "Well there goes a hundred years of history," dryly griped Peter from the helm. The forestay, which plays an integral part in holding up the boat's mast, unwound itself from its fastening at the head of the boat. Peter had some more colorful words at this mishap. "We're on the fuckin' wind! Somebody fix that!" We re-secured it quickly before the mast noticed its absence.

Now, I should mention that *I* was in my element. I was so excited to be sailing a genuine pilot cutter in the precise conditions it had been built for. I had every confidence in Peter too. After all, he knew this boat better than anyone, having himself sailed it to Canada from England years ago. With the knowledge that we were still "operating within specs" I shimmied out to the end of the bowsprit with my camera to capture this incredible ride in photos. The wind continued to build.

Meanwhile, most of the dignitaries on the committee boat were seasick and throwing up from the bad weather, so they went back into the harbor to seek shelter – taking our push boat with them. We finished the race, but there was no one left to witness it.

Without a push boat, we were forced to sail around the southern tip of Vancouver Island to Oak bay, where we could safely anchor under sail. Davey Jones and the pilot had both had quite enough by that point and were happy it was over. As for myself, I'd had a grand day and the experience of a lifetime. Standing on the shore, I wholeheartedly agreed with Peter's comment: "She's so fucking beautiful. You can't help but look back over your shoulder for one last glimpse when you're walking away from her."

I admit to being completely infatuated by *Carlotta*. I pored over photographs of her and immersed myself in the study of Bristol Channel pilot cutters. I kept up regular correspondence with Peter, in the hopes that he was ready to part with her. He had owned her for more than thirty years, so selling her was not something he would come to lightly. *Carlotta* not being available, we embarked on the plan to build our own wooden pilot cutter replica. We worked with a naval architect to draw a design based on the pilot cutters of old. This involved a lot of correspondence back and forth with the designer. Each time a change was made to the plans, the designer would sign off with 'Onwards we go'. Our dream was coming to fruition. It was all so exciting. Jasper would sketch detailed layouts of the future boat's interior, complete with escape hatches and secret compartments. We would aim to build *'Nutmeg'* (named after our milkshakes in Grenada) ourselves to keep the costs lower, and that would fulfill my dream to build a boat as well.

One particular conversation with the designer upset me though. He was concerned that, because we were all cancer survivors, perhaps we should reconsider taking on such a large and lengthy project. Well, as I described previously, this kind of talk only incited me further. I know he had our best interests at heart, but it kind of stung that someone would view the three of us being cancer survivors as some sort of a handicap against our dream. He was worried that a reoccurrence of any of our diseases could affect the possible completion of the project. It all ended up being a moot point anyways, as the project quickly grew exponentially beyond the means of our budget. We had to abandon it.

Around this time, Peter contacted us. He was going to be away the entire summer sailing season, would we like to sail the boat in his absence? We jumped at the opportunity. Soon after this, he decided he was ready to let *Carlotta* go to new owners. He had not used her at all during the previous sailing season. Wooden vessels can deteriorate quickly when not in regular service, and Peter vowed he would never let *Carlotta* come into a deplorable state of ill repair under his ownership. So a price was settled on and the boat was transferred into our names.

When the time came to deliver *Carlotta* home from Cortes Island to Powell River, I called on a group of skilled friends to help. There was literally tons of associated boat gear that had to be brought out of storage ashore and carried down to be stowed aboard the boat. Sails, anchors, interior fittings, tools, lumber, and so much more. The boat had not been sailed for some time, so many interim repairs needed completion to get us home. It helped having friends who were professional shipwrights, ex-boatswains, and seasoned sailors who knew their way around a traditionally rigged boat. Everyone chose a task and we set about like a swarm of bees over *Carlotta*.

After a full day of work, the crew was keen to hoist the mainsail to see what the boat looked like with the sail up at the dock. I argued that it had been a full day, we were all tired, and I was ready for an early night - we could raise the mainsail in the morning. In fact, some of us were so tired we had already staked out the choicest spots on deck and laid out sleeping gear. But they were super eager to raise the sail, and who was I not to reward the efforts of the day with the prospect of seeing the boat spread her wings at the dock? So all hands turned to raising the mainsail. The gaskets holding the furled sail together were cast off and the call to haul away on the halyards was given. The sail didn't get any further than two feet from its resting position before a thousand dead flies and assorted other cadaverous insects rained down from the folds of the sail onto... the open sleeping bags of the crew. After much cursing and sweeping, the bugs were disposed of and we all sat back on the dock and admired the sail - set boldly against the magnificent backdrop of the early night sky. It was a lovely calm evening and the setting sun was lighting the sky in a beautiful swath of oranges and reds. The warm lights from *Carlotta's* interior oil lamps were casting an inviting glow across the mainsail. It was all so charming.

The following day we sailed her home to Powell River, stopping for a night to anchor on the north side of Savary Island. There were not enough bunks on board for everyone so I spent that night sleeping under the stars in the cockpit on deck. Later that night it rained. In the morning, one by one the crew came up on deck carrying a sodden sleeping bag. The decks leaked so badly that somehow I had stayed drier outside than the crew sleeping down below.

Jasper and Barb and I happily moved aboard and sailed the boat for the following year. We kept the boat in Powell River, where Barb and I worked and Jasper attended school. We sailed mainly in the northern reaches of the Strait of Juan de Fuca, journeying to magical spots such as the islands of Hornby, Savary, Texada and Nelson.

Our first cruise together as a family was in the summer of 2004. It was a memorable two-week circumnavigation of Texada Island. The boat was pretty new to us and we were still getting to know the intricacies of her systems. Our first night at anchor was interrupted by a call on

Barb's mobile phone. It was the Wharfinger in Powell River.

"Do you guys intend to return anytime soon? Because, you left your pick-up truck at the top of the dock all day. Both doors are wide open and the keys are still in the ignition." In our excitement to pack and get underway we had completely forgotten about the truck.

Our third night's anchorage on the cruise was to be in Rouse Bay, on Lasqueti Island. This was a very tiny bay with a narrow entrance that could only be accessed during a high tide for a deep draft vessel such as *Carlotta*. We had never been here before, so as we approached the entrance there was a last-minute tense moment in which we questioned whether or not this was indeed Rouse Bay… Also there was the additional exacerbation as to whether we had timed the tide correctly at the entrance. "Time and tide wait for no man" and neither do thirty tons and fifty feet of unforgiving pilot cutter. Chaucer must have been a sailor. We avoided plowing into Lasqueti Island and dropped anchor in the (correct) bay.

After dinner, Jasper and I rowed around the quiet bay together in our wooden dinghy, *Hobbes*. Jasper quoted the *Wind in the Willows:* "There is *nothing* - absolutely *nothing* – half so much worth doing as simply messing about in boats." There was only one other small powerboat anchored here. Aboard it was a lady flamboyantly dressed in a bright orange muumuu. Was she hailing us to come alongside? We obliged. As she spilt her martini here, there and everywhere, she promptly told us we had anchored incorrectly and in a bad location. Then she informed us that we did not know what we were doing. We thanked her for her concern and wished her a good evening. Rowing back to the boat I said to Jasper, "There is *nothing* - like sailing a boat you don't know, into a bay you don't know, and some lady you don't know, tells you that you don't know what you're doing." Jasper giggled at that, and he repeated it back to me many a time for several years following.

One of the complexities of moving *Carlotta* was that she had no internal combustion engine. Originally, of course, she would not have had one when she was built in 1899. Many years later an engine was installed aboard, but Peter had made the decision to once again go without. To be rid of the engine's associated systems and their costs can be a motivating argument for tossing the 'iron jib' over the side. Fuel tanks, batteries, oil, diesel, propellers, and fittings drilled obtrusively into the hull; these all add up quick in the form of money, maintenance, and weight. However, it can come at the high price of stress for the Skipper. You need to be vigilant of the lee shore and the position of the vessel, lest you should be dashed against a breaking shoreline or swept up in a tidal race out of control. If something goes wrong one cannot simply push a button and let the engine solve the problem. Peter had sailed the boat from England without the aid of an auxiliary engine. He had kept her engineless for the past thirty-six years, so I was willing to give it a go too. The tides and currents of British Columbia are strong, not to mention the fickle weather. You needed to be constantly on guard of your surroundings sailing *Carlotta* without an engine here.

Included with *Carlotta* was a twelve-foot long push boat with a twenty-five horsepower gas outboard motor attached to it. This was to be lashed stoutly along *Carlotta's* aft quarter to maneuver the vessel when the wind fell light, or to move her in the sometimes-tight confines of a marina. This method of propulsion was less than ideal; slow, loud, fuel hungry, and heavy helmed. When we were sailing it had to be cast off and towed behind, adding considerable drag and slowing us down. When it was required to be put back into service we were faced with the heavy work of hauling it alongside, jamming several fenders between the two hulls, and then lashing it tightly with four dedicated lines. Then you would leap into it, say a quick prayer to the gods of combustion, and furiously pull the outboard's start cord to bring the beast to life. That was just getting it set up. Adjusting speed and switching into neutral or reverse was another juggling act. Leaping over the side into the pitching push boat and hastily clambering up the side of the hull to regain *Carlotta's* deck was taxing and, depending on the weather and sea conditions at times, downright dangerous. It was pretty much impossible to make any headway at all against anything more than fifteen knots of wind using this system, but if it meant we could propel the boat without violating the integrity of its structure with an internal engine, we were game to give it a try.

The second week into our inaugural family cruise we chose to spend some time anchored in Tribune Bay at Hornby Island. The push boat had greedily guzzled an abominable amount of gas the past week, so I chose to make a run in to shore by myself to refill our empty fuel cans at a gas station not far inland from the beach. There was a strong southerly wind blowing that day and it made for some sizable waves piling up on the beach of Tribune Bay. Timing my landing correctly would be critical to prevent rolling the push boat in the surf (as I had learned from previous experience). I motored in as far as I could, quickly raised the outboard engine into its supportive brackets at the stern, and ran forward with the boat's painter to keep the bow of the boat pointed safely towards the beach. Over the side into waist deep water, I worked fast to pull the heavy boat up to rest on its keel in the sand. The boat was safe, now I needed to unload its contents and find the gas station. I proceeded to cover myself in an elaborate system of ropes and slings to carry the five big gasoline cans up the beach. I was about to start my pilgrimage when I was taken by surprise by a shrill voice in a strangely foreign accent. "Ex-scuze pleeze, Sir. Fleep-floop." I looked up to see a tall tanned man in his early twenties. He had the incredible ripped build of a fitness instructor, and... he was completely naked. I suddenly realized I had landed in '*Little* Tribune Bay', a haven for nude bathers. Again: "Fleep-floop." He was pointing not six feet in front of him. I was confused. What did he want from me? I looked down at what he was pointing to. His flip-flop sandal was floating in the three inches of water between us. Here I was, knackered from my acrobatic surf landing, laden and encumbered to the gills with gas cans, and I was supposed to pick up his sandal? "Um, are you kidding me?" I left him to fish his own sandal out of the brine.

Our summer holiday came to conclusion upon our return to Powell River. It was a busy Saturday afternoon, and the marina was almost full to capacity. Before entering the harbor, we called the Wharfinger and were directed to tie against another vessel just inside the entrance. Barb took up position on *Carlotta's* bow, ready with the dock lines and a pike pole. I would be stationed in the push boat to control our speed. And Jasper – six years old at the time – stood in the cockpit with the enormous five-foot long teak tiller in both hands to control the direction of our outcome. As we came around the end of the breakwater, the boat we had been instructed to tie up against came into view. Oh God, why did it have to be *that* one. It was a multi-million dollar affair, polished to a brilliance beyond bright white, and gleaming in lustrous brass – or was that solid gold? It appeared that fate was upping the ante in our game of docking this boat - considerably. Well, there was no going back as there wasn't the room to turn around. So onwards we went, a six year old on the helm of a fifty-foot long boat that displaces thirty tons and is sporting a twelve-foot long solid fir bowsprit straight out the front like a battering ram. Oh, and a measly twenty-five horsepower outboard to bring this colossus to a stop.

It sounded like a recipe for disaster, but we pulled it off (this time) without a hitch. Thoroughly satisfied by our high degree of seamanship, we stood looking down on *Carlotta* from the elevated deck of the plastic palace, and set about patting each other on the back in praise. There was one thing that had slipped my mind though. It became evident when I looked down between the vessels. Our fenders - bumpers that were positioned between the two hulls, were recycled rubber airplane tires - prone to leaving ugly black skid marks on anything they touched...

Initially, when we bought *Carlotta* we had a pre-purchase survey carried out on her, so we fully understood the condition of the boat. Barb and I knew there would be inevitable large repairs to carry out in the future, but the boat was at the time fully operational. I was somewhat blinded to these repairs by *Carlotta's* beauty. She really is the kind of boat that you can't help but look back over your shoulder for one more glimpse. I think I may have been wearing my rose colored glasses during the pre-purchase survey. Or perhaps more accurately, my thick-lensed rose-colored 'rot-goggles'. After a year of living aboard, we decided to give *Carlotta* some necessary repairs. Also, over the course of time, she had been re-arranged and altered significantly from her original self. We wished to restore her to something in keeping with her original design.

We moved the boat to Finn Bay, next to Lund, just north of Powell River and began a project that led to be an eight-year restoration. There was a small-scale shipyard across from Lund on Sevilla Island that specialized in wooden boats. Bill, the Shipwright from the yard, initially helped me with some of the larger repairs to *Carlotta*. Bill also owned a small house on the island that he rented out during the summer seasons. We moved into the cute, blue shingled, character cottage perched just above the high tide mark. *Carlotta* was at the dock in the bay and the shipyard was a short stroll down a path from the house. It couldn't have been a more idyllic situation. Bill gave me guidance on how to go about repairs on *Carlotta*. I would work part-time for him, honing my skills on other people's boats (and getting paid for it), and then put those skills to use rebuilding *Carlotta*. I was finally realizing my dream to build boats.

We started the restoration by replacing a handful of frames and some of the planking. *Carlotta*, being originally built as a workboat, had massive scantlings. Although she was fifty feet on deck, a lot of her construction was heavier than the one hundred and eleven foot long *Pacific Swift*. Located across Finn bay from us was *Jack's Boatyard*. It had a lift that could *just* handle *Carlotta's* thirty tons. This was where we would replace the frames and planks. The rest of the restoration could take place with the boat in the water at the dock. We would take down the rig and erect a shelter over her entire length. Then we set to gutting the interior. It took several months of deconstruction before we even came close to changing direction by putting some new wood back into her.

The first new piece of construction was to her stern. Sometime in the 1970's the graceful curved counter stern was found to be rotten, so it was cut short by three feet and a flat slab of teak was fastened in its place. In the 1970's the wooden boat movement wasn't as fastidious as it is today. The idea back then was to get your boat fit for sea and go sailing. My very first task would prove to be the trickiest. I had to make sense of multiple curves approaching the stern from all directions, with nothing straight or flat to work from. Using old photographs and carefully running long wooden battens stretched across her hull, I was able to replicate the missing stern. "The hardest part is getting started", and I started with the hardest part.

The list of jobs I took on was enormous. It read like a list for a shipwright's school education: deck beams, stanchions, rudder trunk, covering boards, deck, bulwarks, floors, lining, bulkheads, knightheads, cabin sole, cockpit, Samson posts, and cavels just for a start. The boat consumed huge amounts of new wood. Each of these jobs was a giant project to undertake – largely done singlehanded, by myself. Everything was a chore to bring to the island. Large piles of lumber would be carried down to the shoreline in Lund or the dock across the bay, loaded by hand into a cargo boat, shuttled across to the Sevilla Island dock, and then carried up the ramp to the house or shipyard. More often then not I would time the tide incorrectly and be faced with a steep descent and climb on each end, down and up the ramp of the dock. It was exhausting work, as everything needed for the restoration was immensely big and heavy.

In the basement of the little house, I restored the boat's deck furniture. The skylights and companionway hatch and forward scuttle were stripped and repaired and then each finished with twelve coats of varnish. Also in the basement I rebuilt many of the original fittings of the boat - brass oil lamps were fixed and polished, teak companionway ladders were refreshed, wooden blocks from the rigging were renewed, leather chafe gear was re-stitched and replicated, and the anchor windlass was remanufactured. The boat continued to swallow massive amounts of lumber. Some of this thankfully came as a gift from the previous owner. Peter had earmarked piles of English oak and Burmese teak for *Carlotta* years ago, and squirrelled it away into storage. I searched out local B.C. lumberyards for all the necessary additional timbers. Stacks upon stacks of yellow cedar were acquired. A semi-trailer truckload of Douglas fir was delivered, with thirty-foot long lengths of perfectly clear, tight-grained, air-dried wood for the decks.

I converted the space under the deck of the house into a spar building shop. A thirty-foot long ten by ten beam would become the new main boom. Several other spars needed replacement as well, including a new topmast and a new bowsprit. Each of these was brought down from a four-sided beam, hewn to eight sides, then shaped to sixteen, and finally thirty–two sides, before completion by smoothing them into round poles. Then, they too would receive the multiple coats of varnish to protect them.

Every winter I would reinforce the covered shelter over *Carlotta* so it could withstand the winter storms of British Columbia. Long time resident neighbors in Finn Bay had watched me build the shelter over *Carlotta*. I later learned that they were taking bets as to whether it would survive or not. A bad storm came through one year, knocking down old growth trees in Vancouver's Stanley Park and tearing off a section of the City's BC Place stadium – my tarp stayed on. I remember the wind on that particular day pulsating with the thunderous sound of a train. I had never heard a wind sound like that before, nor do I wish to ever experience it again.

At the same time as the restoration was being undertaken, I studied how to build an Internet website and launched one for *Carlotta*. Once there was a web presence and a contact email, I was soon overwhelmed by correspondence from folks all around the world for whom the boat had played a part in their lives. Relatives of previous owners contacted me with old photographs and stories. They told me of princesses sailing aboard, and of the boat surmounting horrific weather, or how it made remarkably fast passages. There were tales of a porpoise swimming across her swamped foredeck during rough weather. There were incredible accounts relating to her daring survival of the Second World War. Being so old, *Carlotta* had touched the lives of a lot of people. She was a dear object that, to many folks, had represented a time of joy, or deliverance, or an overcoming of hardship.

It was not cheap to haul *Carlotta* at Jack's Boatyard for her annual coat of antifoul bottom paint. I set about building a 'tidal grid' to work around this expense. *Carlotta's* bottom is designed in a fashion that she can sit comfortably on a beach on her keel, supported alongside a pair of pilings. Essentially, a tidal grid operates by positioning a vessel next to those pilings during a high tide. As the tide recedes the boat is left 'high and dry' for maintenance to be conducted until the following tide would refloat her. A tidal grid makes for a cheap, convenient way of accessing a boat's bottom for work – provided you get everything done that you had planned before the sea starts to rise again.

I found a suitable area to build the tidal grid right in front of the house on Sevilla. First I would have to move a few big boulders that were in the way. This would require some ingenuity from Jasper and I. The largest rock was five feet in diameter. At low tide Jasper helped me wrap some ropes around it. Then as the tide came over it, we took a herring skiff – a large flat-bottomed aluminum workboat, and floated over the rock. We grabbed the ropes and secured them tightly to the skiff. As the tide came up it lifted the skiff, which then lifted the attached boulder from its resting spot. We then motored out into the depths of the bay and dropped the boulder to its new home. Jasper loved it. We were like two boys playing with gigantic Tonka toys.

Once the tidal grid's footprint had been cleared, I anchored enormous wooden sleepers into the seabed for the boat's keel to eventually sit upon. The next step was to erect two vertical poles for the boat to support her topside's against. These would prevent a boat on the grid from tipping over as the tide receded. They would be fifty-foot long creosote pilings. I commandeered the help of some friends to get them pointed skyward. There were a few tense seconds between when the pole was hoisted vertical, and the moment where its base was safely socketed home into the beach. Once a piling was upright, it was held in position by four long ropes, an adult at the end of each one maintaining a constant tension. There weren't quite enough adults in the work crew, so we had to enlist some of their children to help. The fate of the project was briefly held in balance by a twelve-year old boy, alone at the end of one of these ropes, the pole teetering precariously above us all. It started to tilt away from him. He found himself suddenly faced with everyone shouting at once, "Pull, Tobijas! Pull!" We all breathed a collective sigh when the two pilings were finally socketed into their cement homes and braced against the beach. Now it was possible to work on the hull of *Carlotta* between tides, without having to arrange and pay for a lift at the yard.

Most of *Carlotta's* restoration was physically backbreaking work to undertake. It was a massive project to mentally contemplate. As long as I stayed focused on a small task at hand right in front of me, I was able to stay sane and not be lost to the stress and anxiety of the years of daunting work spread before me. It helped to be under the tutelage of such a great teacher and Master Shipwright as Bill. He was so open to sharing his art with me. Sure, I learned a lot of boatbuilding skills from him, but even more so, Bill taught me things about life by just being the amazing person he is. Bill was patient and caring and understanding. He is one of the most peaceful and kind persons that I have ever met. I am humbled by him and honored to call him a friend. It is funny to look back on the eight years of restoring *Carlotta* and admit I learned a lot about shipbuilding, but perhaps more importantly, I learned a lot about myself. I learned patience in the face of the broad scope of the project ahead of me. I learned self-awareness from the long days spent in solitude. I learned where my body's physical limits lay. I learned peacefulness; an inner sense of calm from being immersed in the beautiful surroundings of Sevilla Island.

While *Carlotta's* restoration was ongoing, Barb and Jasper and I embraced our time on Sevilla Island. It was a postage stamp-sized island of less than a quarter mile in circumference, with a predominantly rocky shoreline around a low hill with a good covering of large confiners. Sevilla was a charming quintessential gem of a British Columbian island. There was a series of quaint dirt paths and wooden boardwalks that snaked their way around the nine houses and the boat yard. There was one single dock on the protected lee side of the island that the handful of residents commuted back and forth from. The little blue house we rented from Bill was perched right above this dock, facing in toward the shelter of Finn bay. The old house was affectionately known as 'Helen's House', named after Helen Anderson, who was a member of one of the original homesteader families to the Lund area. Helen was long gone, but the urban myths surrounding her remained. One I particularly enjoyed was how she could put a pot of potatoes on the stove to boil, row out into the bay, catch a good sized salmon, and be back in time for the vegetables to be ready.

Sevilla Island was such a special place for us. In the summer we could enjoy a refreshing swim off the dock at the end of the day – all of us laughing and playing in the sunshine. On Friday afternoons the islanders would congregate on the dock to share a beer as they returned home from work. Summer also meant that our garden was in bloom, and walking into the yard you were met with the heavy scents of lavender and hops. In the morning the tweets and twitter of many songbirds greeted you. At night we would sleep on the porch and fall into our dreams under the incredible view of the stars. The evening sky was exceptional as we were so far from any city light pollution.

Life on the island felt a little more isolated during the winter months. For a week each winter it would be cold enough that a sheet of ice formed over the bay, thick enough to make boat passages a challenge. Sometimes rowing home in the dinghy on a winter night we were treated to a magical light show of phosphorescent particles in the water. Jasper would sit in the bow, gazing into the illuminated phosphoresce below, with the magnificent winter night sky of stars wheeling above him, and the twinkling cozy lights of Sevilla Island lost somewhere in between.

We would often lose our electricity due to the winter storms, sometimes for a week in duration. The house was heated with a woodstove, which we kept going constantly from September to March. It was a fight to keep the house warm during this time, it being so old and lightly insulated. Jasper would position himself directly in front of the woodstove's glass door with his current book, basking in the hot orange glow of heat. Wood to feed that stove did not come easy. It had to be brought by boat from Lund and involved several trips of carrying it up and down the beach on both ends, followed by chopping and stacking it. By the time you were finished you were too hot to want to light a fire. Jasper and I would also cruise the nearby beaches of the Copeland islands for any recent windfall we could salvage. Once we spied a suitable piece we would get to work with a chainsaw and tow the log home to add to our stash of firewood.

We were remote enough that the odd black bear or cougar would visit the island. We had to keep Jasper carefully within our sights for a two-week period when a cougar temporarily took up residence under our neighbor's porch. At times a bear would frequent the island. One morning we watched one swim across the bay and disappear into the trees. Later that week we witnessed it prying the wooden siding, nails and all, off an outbuilding next to our house. This was a stoutly built shed that was being stripped of its walls as effortlessly as you or I peel a ripe banana. The screech of metal nails being pulled out of breaking boards is not a comforting sound to hear when you've just settled in for the night. We scared him away by banging some pots and pans.

Every morning Barb and Jasper would row our little wooden rowboat *'Hobbes'* a short distance into Finn Bay, and then drive the thirty minutes into Powell River for school and work. You would think anyone commuting by rowboat an anomaly, but there were actually three separate islanders that rowed in to shore each day. I would go to work at the yard, either on a client's boat or *Carlotta*. In the late afternoon I'd venture into Lund to pick up Jasper from the school bus. After securing my work skiff to the Lund gas dock I'd trudge up the road above the hamlet to where the school bus would drop him off. Friday afternoons were special. We would stop in at the Lund General Store for two Jones Sodas and a bag of Hawkins Cheezies, or if it was raining and cold out we'd go sit in Nancy's Bakery with a cup of hot chocolate while Jasper pored over Nancy's selection of National Geographic magazines.

Jasper developed quite a reputation up and down the Sunshine Coast. Everyone knew Jasper. If I met someone new in my community it was always "*Oh!* You're *Jasper's* dad." This was partly because he was participating in so many extra curricular activities in the community. He was involved in everything all over town: choir, piano,

T-ball, soccer, music, sailing, and swim club - the list of his interests was endless! And being such an animated, charismatic, outgoing person, he made many good friends.

He was a popular guy. He was elected as his school's Student President. His school offered a second language program, and he began lessons in Tla'amin, the local first nation band's dialect. His teacher nicknamed him X'wup X'wup, Tla'amin for hummingbird, as Jasper moved and lived at a speed that was hard to comprehend. It was hard to keep up with him. A group of Jasper's schoolmates teamed together for a competition between schools all over North America called *'Destination Imagination'*. The premise was that each group would quickly form an impromptu skit using key phrases, historical figures, and assorted situations within a short time frame. You had to be quick on your feet, have a strong knowledge of history, and be able to rally your team together to perform the skit – all things right up Jasper's alley. His team ended up winning the regional and provincial competitions, and travelled together to the global finals in Knoxville, Tennessee.

Jasper and Barb thought a dog would be a good addition to our family. The problem was that I had a minor allergic reaction to dog hair. They researched Scottish Border Terriers: a breed with a hypoallergenic wire coat, and small enough to live aboard a boat. We drove down to a respectable breeder in Chemainus on Vancouver Island to have a look at them. Jasper and Barb had no intention to buy a dog that day, and I certainly had not been convinced yet. On the trip there I repeatedly reminded them that we were only looking. We were shown the latest litter. One puppy in the pen was leaping back and forth with an abundance of energy compared to the rest. This energetic dog caught my attention. Then I realized it only had one eye. The breeder explained that the mother had mistakenly damaged it the day the puppy was born. I felt a one-eyed kinship with this beast, and (surprisingly?) we were soon homeward bound with a new addition to our family: Pippa.

The next day Barb and Jasper went to Powell River on their daily commute and they left me in charge of the dog. Pippa and I went out to work on the dock next to *Carlotta*. Bill went by in his motorboat and gave us a friendly wave. Pippa climbed up and perched herself on the railing of the dock facing his boat. Was she planning to jump in to pursue him? Could she even swim? I was too far away to bridge the distance and grab her. I had just finished mouthing the words "No... you *wouldn't*." when she leapt from the railing, belly flopped into the cold water, and sank out of sight. "Oh my God, I've killed the dog on the very first day of ownership!" She reappeared at the surface and began dog-paddling towards Bill's boat, which was now fast disappearing out of the bay. "Pippa! Pippa! Pippa! Pippa!" I called. Could she even know her name at this stage? Yes. She turned around. She did know her name. I was so relieved. But now she was wet and shivering with cold. We returned to the house where I dried her off and wrapped her in a warm blanket next to the woodstove.

That same week, Pippa and I came home to the house for lunch. I left her outside while I went in to fix myself some food. I remember there was not much to eat in the house that day. I would have to suffice with a cup of tea and a measly cheese sandwich. I got curious as to what Pippa was up to. I peered out the kitchen window and low and behold, she was eating an entire chicken dinner from the contents of a take-a-way package. We were on a remote isolated island - where on earth did she get that? Trust the dog to find a better meal than I'd get.

Jasper had free run of Sevilla Island and he now had the dog as a partner in his adventures. He would manufacture a wooden sword and head off in his lifejacket and rubber boots to explore with Pippa. He and I built a hidden bunker into the side of a hill in the middle of the island, from where he could spy out with binoculars over the surrounding seas and spot all of the comings and goings. A boy living on an island naturally takes to learning how to row. He became an expert at sculling *Hobbes* - rowing it by standing in the stern and propelling it with a one-handed motion using a single oar. He soon became confident enough to row into Finn bay on his own to pick up a friend from school to play.

Jasper showed an early interest in music. He enjoyed singing and had a great voice for it, even when he was a toddler. He took up piano lessons and developed a love for jazz music in particular. He loved singing, so he joined the local boys choir too. He played a multitude of instruments including the trombone, guitar, ukulele, and... tuba. Because Jasper had skipped ahead in school, he was smaller than his classmates. Why is it the smallest kid in the school orchestra always ends up with the largest instrument? It was hilarious seeing him touting around this giant tuba. It was quite the sight when he and Barb would pile into *Hobbes* with it for the morning commutes.

Jasper got his first job at the library in Powell River as a Page. He would re-shelve library books and perform other errands. His interview for the position included a 'height test' to see if he could reach the top shelf. He was very proud of his job and made many friends with the staff. With his love of books it really was the perfect fit for him.

Jasper formed a close friendship with Zach, a boy who lived half way between Lund and Powell River. Zach's father worked in Finn Bay, so Zach and Jasper were able to see a lot of each other. Zach was always a very happy and friendly chap, and wow, could he talk the ears off a brass monkey. It was nonstop chatter between the two of them. An exchange with Jasper could leave folks scratching their heads, flabbergasted by his vocabulary, while Zach seemed able to talk at twice the speed of an auctioneer.

Any Saturday morning, despite the fact they'd been up for most of the previous night, I could walk into the kitchen and find Zach already operating at 110 percent, busy in the process of flipping pancakes. Jasper would be sitting at the kitchen table in front of a plate of untouched flapjacks, distracted with his nose right up against the screen of his laptop.

"Heyyyy, Papa. Check out this rocket I built on K.S.P. (Kerbal Space Program). It's a three-stage Mk-1 with ion propulsion and twin J-404 'Panther' afterburning turbofans. Xenon fuel tanks, Papa! *Three hours* at full thrust! That's enough tangential speed to perform a radial-out burn to slow the rocket with aerobrakes and a lowered periapsis. It'll be sub-orbital and eventually collide with the planet, but oh well... the crew are just Kerbals. Isn't that cool, Papa?"

"Huh?" I rub the sleep from my eyes. "Oh. Yeah. Sure. Kerbals..."

"Oh! Stephen! I-made-you-some-pancakes-and-can-Jasper-and-I-please-have-a-sleepover-again-cause-we're-going-out-on-Gone-Bananas-to-the-Copeland-Islands-and-my-Mom-and-Dad-and-Nana-are-going-and-we're-going-to-bring-the-Gameboys-and-have-a-fire-on-the-beach-with-smokies-and-go-swimming-today!" He takes a breath. "Oh-and-goodmorning-Stephen! Goooooood morning, Barb."

Reeling, I would contemplate going straight back to bed.

Between the two of them, a conversation was like four people talking at once. Zach and Jasper grew to be as close as brothers. Zach's family owned a twenty-foot-long, bright yellow catamaran: *'Gone Bananas'*. On weekends they would come by the Sevilla Island dock to pick Jasper up. Jasper would spend the weekend with them exploring all the nooks and crannies of the nearby Copeland Islands: renaming all the bays there, enjoying campfires ashore, and swimming and playing with Zach. Jasper's childhood really was the stuff of boyhood dreams, of the same vein in many ways as my childhood.

It came as a surprise to me when my Dad passed away in the winter of 2007. Dad had polycystic kidney disease. He had it his entire life, but it wasn't until then that it effectively debilitated him. He chose to go on an at-home dialysis machine, as travelling back and forth to the hospital in Nanaimo was taxing on him and Mom. Dad passed away suddenly from an aneurism that January. I was crushed. I had just seen him the week before and he seemed fine. I had never lost anyone so close to me.

I went to visit Mom to be with her. That night I went outside into the garden. I sat on a wooden tree-swing suspended on long ropes between two big cedars. Dad had built this swing. It was just like a tree swing he built on our acreage in Pine Valley. Dad would push me on that one when I was young. "Do an under-push Dad!" I would call out, and he would push and run and disappear underneath me. Now, this swing seemed all that more special to me. Actually, Barb and I had our wedding photos taken on it. I remember visiting Dad just after he had finished building this one. He had laughed when I undid the bulbous rope knots he had tied, and in their place I'd tucked two proper shipshape rope splices. He beamed at me with a smile and a look of fascination that I could do such a feat so effortlessly. He had always been so proud of me. Now he was gone forever. I sat on the swing, and I cried.

CHAPTER ELEVEN

LOW BLOW TO THE GUT

It had been seven years since we had begun, and now *Carlotta's* restoration was complete. This called for a celebration. We called it a 'Re-Birthday Party' and everyone was invited. The party would include a giant slab cake, the Lund Shanty-men singers, and a Celtic fiddle band that Barb played in. We moved *Carlotta* to the Lund Hotel dock for the day. Folks came from up and down the coast to join in the fun. In fact, there were so many people gathered on the dock that it started sinking under the strain. Speeches were made, music was played, cake was eaten, and everyone got a chance to take a tour through the newly restored boat. A happy day indeed.

Many people had gotten wind of the project we had taken on and would visit Finn Bay to have a look. We made lots of new friends this way. Folks journeyed from afar to witness *Carlotta's* rebuild. That summer we were able to complete the rigging and go for our first sail since the restoration. Joining us on board for that inaugural sail was a visitor from England whose father had sailed the boat in the 1950's and 1960's. It was quite a treat to hear his old stories. He was so delighted to play a part in the boat's first return to sail, and for the occasion he wore his father's old, original sailing smock too.

We enjoyed sailing *Carlotta* on several memorable trips. Jasper's thirteenth birthday party was a sleepover aboard with friends. It included swimming, sailing, pizza and cake. It was wonderful to see his young friends so keen to take a hand in sailing the boat. They were excited to be given the chance to raise and trim sails, haul up the anchor, or take a turn at the helm. They were eager to try rowing *Carlotta* too. When the wind fell away to nothing and the sea was calm we would use two gigantic eighteen-foot-long wooden oars to (slowly) pull *Carlotta* along. Once you got her moving, rowing was actually quite easy and satisfying work. The boat still didn't have an engine, but we had thoughts of installing one in the not-too-distant future. When the sails were dropped and I had to rely on the use of the underpowered push-boat to maneuver *Carlotta's* thirty tons, it was a real test of my sanity.

The time came to move aboard. It should have been a joyous and exciting time. Instead, I began experiencing incredible bouts of stress and anxiety. The keenly anticipated move out of the Sevilla Island house and onto the boat, coupled with coming to terms that the project was over, and the realization that my job at the shipyard was finishing, all took a toll on me in the form of significant anxiety. Everything became a source of stress to me. One afternoon it became too much and I suffered a significant panic attack. I saw a doctor and he prescribed antidepressants and anti-anxiety medication.

We moved out of the little blue house and into our new home. All of us really enjoyed finally being aboard her. She was so new and clean and smelled wonderful down below. It was October, and Thanksgiving Day Barb cooked us turkey with all the fixings on our woodstove in the galley. Our first few weeks living aboard were all so cozy.

My mind had eased somewhat now that we were living aboard, but I had started experiencing sharp stomach pains. I suspected it was an ulcer as a result of all the worrying I had been doing of late. With my history of cancer I couldn't be too careful, so I was booked for a gastroscopy – a procedure under anesthetic in which they send a scope down your throat to have a look around. Jasper was feeling ill that week too. He had been throwing up and having bad headaches. We thought the worst: it might be meningitis. Twice we took him to the Powell River hospital. Perhaps he was having migraines? They did a CAT scan and sent the results to Dr. Strahlendorf in Vancouver.

The next day I was in a dressing gown in the surgery ward readying for the gastroscopy, when Barb got word back from Dr. Strahlendorf; she would like us to make the trip to the B.C. Children's hospital to discuss the results of the CAT scan. Should I call off my procedure? No, Barb and I decided, I should get this resolved so we could be fully ready to tackle whatever was going on with Jasper.

It was all a whirlwind from that point on. I awoke from the surgery. There were signs that an ulcer had been present, but it was now healing. Good. Although, we didn't get time to fully process this positive news. We had to get to Vancouver as soon as possible.

It was on Tuesday, November 22, 2011 when we tore off to catch the next ferry to Vancouver. We had one change of clothes each. We left Pippa and *Carlotta* in the care of some friends, and we headed off toward the unknown.

CHAPTER TWELVE

INTO THE FIRE

We arrived in Vancouver at the B.C. Children's Hospital and were ushered straight into a meeting with Dr. Strahlendorf. When the words 'mass' and 'anomaly' were mentioned, the room began to spin. I was going to pass out if I didn't get horizontal in a hurry. I was urged to stretch out on an examination table that was pressed up against a wall in the office. I was hit by far too many sensations at once; the crisp, crinkling sound of the paper covering the table I slumped into, my heavy body encumbered by the wet winter boots and Pea coat I was still wearing; the nauseating sterile smells of bleached floors and filtered air; the piercing bright fluorescent lights; that background sound of the hospital's air-conditioning system, like an ever-present quiet storm brooding. "This *can't* be happening," I thought. A nurse passed me a cold glass of water. I sat up and took a sip, drew a deep breath, and lay back down to regain my bearings. Granted, I was still recovering from surgery, but how ironic that Jasper was the patient, yet I was the one needing the medical attention. Jasper took the news bravely. He expressed his worries about missing school and his new job at the library as a Page. Barb remained levelheaded and confident. She had lots of questions for the doctor.

We were thrust into a series of tests and procedures. Jasper was scheduled for an immediate MRI scan to get a clear picture of what we were dealing with. There was very little time for Barb and I to process the news of his diagnosis. We launched back into our roles as parents of a child with cancer, guiding and caring for him. We stood by him while he was poked, prodded, scanned, and inspected. Before the week's end, he had surgery on his brain, to relieve pressure and obtain a biopsy.

We had been thrown back into the familiar fires of the Children's Hospital. The last days of November passed rapidly. Yes, the initial news was bad, but we were given a treatment plan that seemed logical and hopeful.

Being admitted to hospital as a long-term patient was a different experience from our previous visits to day surgery, when Jasper was an infant. Over the past years of check-ups we had become familiar with the staff of nurses, anesthetists, and doctors of day surgery. Now, we would have an entire team working with us, comprised of nurses and doctors of various specialties; a psychologist, social workers, and a host of music, sport, and diet therapists. Our visits to the hospital used to be limited to a route between the day surgery ward and the cafeteria, with an annual visit to the oncology ward. We were now faced with crossing back and forth from one far end of the hospital complex to the other, with regular stops to all the departments in between; audiology for a hearing test, then upstairs and across the ped-way to have blood drawn, radiology for an x-ray, then return to oncology for a chemo cocktail or blood transfusion. Any number of unscheduled additional tests or procedures could be thrown into the mix at the last minute. It was exhausting and taxing on us all. We grew accustomed to the system of checking-in to any department and then settling in to the purgatory of a waiting room. As an admitted patient, Jasper was tagged with a personal hospital identification number. He soon memorized the number from his wrist bracelet. He would be quick to ring off the code just before a nurse was about to confirm his identity for taking blood, or to a technician who was about to check his details against a chart. This would take them by surprise. "1072066." He sounded like a Stormtrooper checking in for duty.

In the middle of December Barb and I were able to obtain a room at the Ronald McDonald House, however, Jasper remained in the hospital until January. When we came to the house with Jasper as a baby we were in one day and out the next, so we didn't connect with the staff or other families. Our family was now in need of extended stays here. The house became a sanctuary of love for us.

Ronald McDonald House provided a safe, economical, clean, friendly environment to stay at while in Vancouver.

It was ideally situated close to the hospital. Cancer patients with a compromised immune system have strict guidelines of cleanliness to adhere to, and the Ronald McDonald House maintained these high standards. The fridges were kept stocked with donated food, and volunteers occasionally made meals for the families. The house was furnished in the spirit of an actual home, a welcome place to be when compared to the institutional surroundings of the hospital.

Jasper, Barb and I were comfortable at the house. We all made close friendships there. It was a special place. Jasper could play and interact with other kids there, or he could escape on his own with a book. Barb and I could share experiences and feelings amongst other parents who were on a similar journey. It provided us with a real home away from the hospital.

During our first week at the house, I cried for the first time since my dad had passed away. Late one night, Barb and I were alone in the room. Barb had just shut off the lights in preparation for bed. A full moon was beaming through the window, casting the room in a blue light. As I stood looking out at the dark autumn night, my mind began to race with worry.

"Are we going to lose him?" I asked. There was trepidation in my wavering voice. I felt that I could cry, but I was worried that I may wake or disturb other families in the adjoining rooms if I did so. Fear continued to spread over me. I fought back an outburst, trying to remain composed.

Barb approached and put her arms around me. I slumped forward and let it all go, weeping aloud and uncontrolled. "Are we going to lose him? I don't want to lose my son! I can't live without my son…" I sobbed. I didn't care anymore if someone heard me wailing. I cried until there was nothing left. I felt drained and exhausted. I did my best to find my breath.

I had tried so hard to hold back my tears because I didn't want to wake anyone. It turns out that's okay at this house; because the folks down the hall completely understand. Those families are all in crisis too.

When you're in crisis, sometimes the best thing to do is to put your head down and push on. Winston Churchill said, "If you're going through hell, keep going." But for how long were we to endure this? With the swift passing of time, days turned to weeks, and then to months. When would we see home again?

We just kept going.

CHAPTER THIRTEEN

ONWARDS WE GO…

Many of my journal entries are signed off with 'Onwards we go…' I adopted the phrase as it harkens back to the suggestion that I should avoid building *Nutmeg* due to our shaky past health history. I would take its intention and spin it on its ear – to say *yes, we will* do this, and *we can* overcome. It would prove to be my anthem during Jasper's treatment. It empowered me to keep going, to not give up despite adversity and odds. It instilled hope, and Lord knows, I needed something hopeful sounding at the end of a lot of these entries.

Monday, January 30, 2012 at 6:32pm

Barb wrote this latest update: Hello Everyone, I thought I would send an update even though our past little while has been blissfully uneventful from a medical perspective. We have been out of the hospital for about ten days now and staying at the Accent Inn. This is because we are all getting over colds, which prevent us from staying at the Ronald McDonald House. We hope to get back there on Tuesday or Wednesday this week. In the meantime the Accent Inn in Richmond is a nice place to land (Provincial health care is paying). This is where we stayed when first diagnosed in November. We are doing a lot of catching up on sleep, eating, watching TV, playing video games and guitar and violin, doing homework, building websites and generally hangin'. Jasper has been eating and gained some weight - which is great. His appetite is now normal and growing, although some food smells can still make him nauseous. Jasper has connected with friends from home online and through gaming. Zach and his father came to visit last week and we all went to the BC Museum of Anthropology. They have a beautiful collection and Jasper and I had never been there before. We will definitely visit again. My parents were also here for a visit and we were able to connect with some Vancouver area friends too. Last Saturday Jasper wanted to go to the central branch of the Vancouver library, which is modeled after the Coliseum in Rome. Jasper and Opa were in their element, overcome by books and architecture at the same time. He got a 'BC One' Library Card and checked out a stack of novels. Another highlight for Jasper was going to the Vancouver Film School's Video Game Design Expo last Sunday where he attended a few sessions about game design and game storytelling and saw some of the games in development by students. Other than colds, the general reason for the break was that Jasper's blood counts have to rise in order for him to have chemo on Tuesday. This round of chemo will be a "mini" round using only one of the chemo drugs in order to send him through the cycle that produces stem cells. We were not able to collect any the last round and they are necessary for the chemo he will be having in March-May. This mini-round should not make him feel as sick. They think he might be able to be discharged after about two days. This is great because we are looking forward to him being in good spirits for the skate on Friday where we will 'Skype' in. The test run with Skype this week was successful and we are excited about seeing our friends in the community. It still seems weird that we left Powell River with about three hours notice and haven't been back... Tomorrow we are thinking of going downtown to 'Phat Bagel' and maybe catch a matinee (Monday matinees have not so many of the flu-ridden hordes attending that we have to keep Jasper away from!). Today we are hoping to go to the beach somewhere - Jasper misses the birds and the ocean. - Barb

Wednesday, February 1, 2012 at 11:13pm

Just finished this 'mini' cycle of chemo. All is going as expected. Unfortunately we got put in room number one on the ward - it's the window-less one painted pale yellow and has creepy looking insects stenciled on the ceiling. Patients around here have affectionately named it 'The Dungeon'. The usual nausea and lack of appetite is present for Jasper, and the minimal sleep pattern for all three of us. This 'mini' two-day chemo cycle will bring his blood counts down, then when they start to climb the hope is to catch the window of opportunity and harvest Jasper's stem cells. This would happen next week. It's a big loud machine that hooks up to his centerline port in his chest and takes a full day. The collected stem cells are used later on to help him bounce back from the heavy aggressive doses of chemo they have planned for him. Onwards we go...

Thursday, February 9, 2012 at 9:27am

No stem cell harvest today. Instead he gets a four-hour hemoglobin transfusion as his blood counts are starting to crash. He's sleepy and sore.

Friday, February 10, 2012 at 10:43am

Stem cells anyone? Jasper is on the stem cell harvesting machine for about ten hours today.

Monday, February 13, 2012 at 3:25pm

I'm downtown waiting for Jasper & Barb to come out of a movie. I'm sitting having a 'Japa-dog' when three movie stars stroll up to order. The paparazzi were shooting photos of them. I don't know who they were, but look for me in TMZ magazine. I'm the guy in the background with mustard all over his face having a conversation with a crow that's after my hot dog.

Tuesday, February 14, 2012 at 8:14am

Back in the chemo circus again today...

Monday, February 20, 2012 at 9:07am

Despite waking up with the beginnings of a cold this morning, blood counts are high enough so Jasper will start chemo today in isolation. Also an X-ray is scheduled for a freaky bone spur on his hand.

Thursday, February 23, 2012 at 2:46pm

Chemo cycle number three of six is over in record time for Jasper at just four days. We are discharged until Tuesday! He had minimal nausea and a healthy appetite this time. He's a strong courageous fighter.

Wednesday, February 29, 2012 at 10:25pm

Jasper got a fever tonight so he was admitted back into hospital. We went thru Emergency where there must have been a hundred kids waiting. Nurses say it's a crazy busy night; everything from pneumonia to getting hit in the head with a baseball bat. Jasper bypassed them all and went straight in. His temperature went up to 39.5. He's on antibiotics now and we're headed up to the last room on floor 2b.

Thursday, March 1, 2012 at 11:39am

This morning's blood work came back positive for infection. So another antibiotic has been added to the mix in his i-v. Unfortunately it also comes with a ten-day stay in hospital.

Monday, March 5, 2012 at 7:01pm

Another transfusion of platelets today. Yesterday was a red blood cell transfusion. We might have to try collecting more stem cells in the next few days. An MRI is scheduled for the 15th, which will give another look at where we stand with the tumor. We're out on a pass for the evening and are going out for dinner as a family. Onwards we go...

CHAPTER FOURTEEN

PRAY FOR PLATELETS

The level of duress Barb and I had been under was off the charts. I would put my head down and just confront things as they were thrown at us. Sometimes everything was such a blur. Running errands around Vancouver I would lose myself in my racing mind and wake up in traffic wondering where I was and how I'd gotten there. Whoa! I'm driving a car down Cambie Street! I could completely blank out. Barb could relate to this, as she had done the same thing.

Barb was such a positive pillar of hope. When we were going through a particularly bad day or confronted by a hardship, Barb would be the encouraging one to see the glass half full. Jasper and I used to tease her about it, making reference to a lyric from Billy Joel's song 'Pressure' about *Peter Pan* advice. Jasper and I would smile at each other and then sing this to her, putting particular emphasis on the cheery elf's name. Barb was our Peter Pan – always hopeful and seeing the bright side, and she was Jasper's best health care advocate. If a nurse asked us for information about medication dosage, Jasper and I could rely on Barb to know the intricate details. If a doctor was explaining a procedure to us, Barb was the one to ask questions and speak out on our behalf. Her biology degree really came into play here. She kept track of everything. She held our family together. If I was Jasper's assigned 'Public Relations Manager', than Barb was his... well, I suppose the ultimate title is *'Mother'*. And what an excellent mother she was.

Barb and I weren't alone though. It is amazing to see where support can come from in times of crisis. Some folks I would have thought would be there for us disappeared completely into the woodwork. Others unexpectedly came forth with all manner of help. It can be a surprise to see who of your friends and family actually step up to the plate. Our family friend Chad was the absolute shining example of a real hero. Chad went above and beyond. He lived and worked in Sidney on Vancouver Island. On so many weekends he would walk onto the ferry (a two hour voyage) and then ride the bus into the city to come and visit us in the hospital or at the Ronald McDonald House. Jasper got to depend on his weekly visits. Barb and I could confidently leave Jasper in Chad's care if we needed to get away for a break. We could confide in Chad. He became another member of our family really.

Jasper and Chad had a special relationship. Chad was kind and understanding and a really good friend to Jasper.

They could play and laugh, or have a serious conversation together. Jasper and I would often take turns at teasing Chad, and a lot of jokes and rubs were at his expense. But Chad was always such a good sport about it. I think he knew Jasper's teasing was an outlet for release, and as a result, Chad provided endless opportunity for banter. A common theme was his early model mobile phone. Chad was constantly at odds trying to get this phone to work properly. It always had some issue or another wrong with it. Jasper liked his tech to be cutting edge and would mock Chad over his "Ancient device!" He would razz him it was "Old enough to be gaff-rigged!" Another easy target of ridicule was Chad's childhood love for the television program 'H.R. Puff n' Stuff'. Chad's descriptions of this oddly twisted 1970's children's show could make Jasper laugh like a sea lion.

Friday, March 9, 2012 at 8:42am

Update from Barb: Jasper had chemotherapy on the twentieth of February and it was one of the shortest hospital stays yet. Jasper ate and drank well throughout and we were allowed to go home on day four! He had been feeling typically rotten since, but felt very at home at Ronald McDonald House where he could cook favorite foods and just relax in a real bed or on a good couch. That weekend we were basically all by ourselves at Ronald McDonald House and they hosted an Oscar party so we invited our friends! The Wolferstans, Chad, the Sepkowskis (with Pippa!) and Mark all came for pizza and we dressed up as movie stars. It was so much fun to have everyone in the same house and to spend some good quality time with Pippa. We have such awesome friends. Stephen and I were just actually starting to talk about maybe making a quick trip home when, on Wednesday last week, Jasper "spiked" a fever. We called the oncologist and she said to come in right away. Boy, were we all of a sudden glad that we were not in Powell River where we would have been basically stuck until the following day. With no white blood cells, Jasper's fever climbed rapidly and they had him on i-v antibiotics within the hour. We were also given priority treatment in an emergency room that must have had more than 100 people in it. Although everyone likes to complain about our medical system, especially wait times, we are always so impressed and grateful for the fast and expert treatment we get when it really counts. It turns out that Jasper had a strep A infection - from his own body again - but within a day it had disappeared from his bloodstream. Unfortunately the 10-day course of intravenous antibiotics means staying attached to the hospital, but Jasper has been out on a "pass" a few times with friends Zach, and then Jessica and Natasha. The past few days, however, Jasper has had some sores and swelling and pain and so he is getting a self-administer morphine machine today which should make him comfortable until this passes. Last time it took two to three days to subside. If all goes well, we may get discharged on Monday. We have our next MRI on Thursday the 15th of March. Everybody start crossing fingers! We are feeling confident that the chemo is working and are hopeful that the tumor is gone. After that it's three more rounds of chemo. At this point we are basically just over half way through the treatment plan. Today Stephen is spending a day with a friend and I am keeping Jasper company. We have lots of visitors popping in over the next couple of weeks - which is great. It always makes the time pass faster. - Barb

Saturday, March 10, 2012 at 9:10pm

Rough evening. He has a fever of 40.5 degrees with shakes and nausea and alarming blood pressures. He's on three antibiotics, three big painkillers, and a variety of other medications. He's really fighting with this latest infection. Also, his counts are low so he'll be getting a platelet transfusion tonight. He's finally drifting off to sleep now.

Sunday, March 11, 2012 at 8:42pm

Jasper's doing better now. No fever today! He continues to fight the latest infection.

Wednesday, March 14, 2012 at 10:41pm

Tomorrow at 12:15 is an MRI scan to see where we stand on the chemotherapy progress. We'll have some results of the scan in the afternoon. Antibiotics are doing their job and Jasper's infections are clearing up. He's not in so much pain anymore so painkillers are being reduced slowly. He's sleepy and sore and isn't able to do much during his day. Good news: his blood counts are beginning to show signs of trending upwards. He's eating and drinking really well and has kept his weight on during this past cycle. Every day he grows stronger.

Thursday, March 15, 2012 at 2:51pm

Good news! The MRI shows the tumor is a thousand percent better than when we began treatment. It continues to shrink, but two more cycles of chemo are necessary. There is still no need for surgery, and radiation is still being discussed.

Friday, March 16, 2012 at 8:26am

Update from Barb: Today we had another MRI to gauge the progress on tumor reduction and the results were excellent. The tumor has shrunk again significantly and borders of the tumor have gotten much thinner (which makes it easier for the chemo to get at it). Our oncologist actually said that the situation is a thousand times better than when we were first admitted and much better than she even dared to hope. This latest look allows the team to fine tune the rest of Jasper's treatment schedule. We will only have 2 more rounds of chemotherapy... the first much like what we've been doing so far, and the last a mega-dose with a stem cell rescue. This is good because, in general, Jasper has really struggled between chemo rounds with infections - and so one less round is welcome! Once again they have confirmed that no surgery is necessary, but after the next round of chemo they will discuss the possibility of radiation with the 'Tumor Board'. Let's hope that the next round eliminates all tumor material and that radiation won't be necessary!

Although the news was great today - it was a difficult day. Jasper's infections and fever seem to be under control, but his blood counts are not coming up as fast as we all would like, and he is still experiencing episodes of pain which are heartbreaking and leave us all feeling exhausted. He has had a lot of morphine and the concern now is weaning him off of it with as few side effects as possible. This makes the ongoing pain management even more difficult. I hope we only have a few more days of this struggle for him. While his blood counts begin to recover over the next few days, they will look for stem cells again to get a 'backup' supply if possible. This may be used to help him recover quicker in the next round, as his bone marrow appears to be getting very tired... We have had many visitors recently and more to come in the next two weeks. We have also had many, many well wishes by email and we are passing them all on to Jasper. - Barb

Thursday, March 22, 2012 at 8:12am

Jasper's discharged from the Hospital. Next cycle of chemo starts Tuesday the 27th.

Monday, March 26, 2012 at 1:14pm

Blood counts are too low so chemo is delayed until Friday. That means Oma and Opa take us to an East Indian buffet lunch. So we stuff ourselves and then head to the 'Hunger Games' movie!

Tuesday, April 3, 2012 at 7:18am

Jasper's counts are too low to start chemo so it has been delayed until next Tuesday.

Wednesday, April 4, 2012 at 5:44pm

We went home to Powell River for 24 hours. Excellent! Had a great time and look forward to getting back home again soon. Best part? I took Jasper out for a night ride on a friend's motorcycle while we were there.

Monday, April 19, 2012 at 3:50pm

Jasper's bald head has opened many doors. Today it actually got us out of a speeding ticket!

Tuesday, April 10, 2012 at 2:09pm

Jasper's counts are still too low to start chemo. We will try again Thursday.

Tuesday, April 10, 2012 at 4:18pm

An update from Barb: Happy Belated Easter. Unfortunately Jasper's bone marrow has still not recovered from his last chemotherapy and so the next round continues to get delayed. It has now been fifty-two days since his last treatment and, although his white cell count is basically there, his platelets fell below threshold today and we were not able to begin. We will go back on Thursday to check again - so everybody think/pray "platelets"! The length of his recovery from this last chemo has our oncologist a little worried about how well he can recover from continued treatment - especially since we were only able to collect the bare minimum of stem cells. She will be reducing the dosage of his next treatment slightly to help the situation. On Thursday she takes his case to the Tumor Board for a recommendation on radiation or not. It's a fine balance...until now we have really been trying to avoid radiation because of the risk of future cancer, but now we may have to look at it from a different angle. A little bit of radiation might be ultimately more effective treatment and less risky to Jasper's immediate health than two more rounds of intense chemo. Although the Tumor Board will make a recommendation, the final decision will not be made until the MRI results that follow this round of chemo that's coming up. This latest delay has thrown us all a little off... Jasper is noting that his hair is starting to grow back, and worries a little about whether the tumor will also grow - but we have been assured that these two things are not connected. It's a very strange place to be - disappointed that chemo hasn't started. It's partially spring fever I think - we are impatient to be done with treatment and start enjoying the weather. In the meantime we have to be thankful for his growing health. When he starts treatment he will be stronger than he has been in a very long time. He has gained almost a kilogram since last week and is looking well. He is eating and drinking and singing and dancing and playing piano and racing remote control cars and generally full of energy. We've had an eventful week. A couple of families we had grown close to at the Ronald McDonald House went home basically for good. One will return for treatment on a once-a-month basis, but it was a little hard to say goodbye. Jasper is hoping to meet up with them again at Camp Goodtimes this summer. We made a short trip home (for Jasper and Stephen, just 24 hours). This was awesome. We live in a beautiful spot and we are definitely eager to get back to it. Jasper kept his visiting to a minimum for this trip, as he was anxious about being overwhelmed. In the end it was just right and he topped off the day with a ride on the back of a motorcycle! He is thinking he will do another one-day visit after the next round of chemo if the opportunity presents. Although the boys stayed only one day, I stayed for three and got lots of quality time in with the Sepkowski's and Pippa. I even got a motorcycle lesson from Tobijas. The weather was beautiful and I walked everywhere. I also connected briefly with work and spent some time on *Carlotta* - she is doing just fine and we were relieved to see things were all warm and dry down below. Easter at the Ronald McDonald House was festive with Jasper helping to hide eggs for the hunt, a great ham dinner, and two giant chocolate bunnies. In the past weeks we have had visits from my family as well as Stephen's mom, and seen good friends Esther, Chad and Andy. Over spring break we had visits from Austin and Joe and Zach. We've had a chance to have some nice dinners out, picnicked by the arrival runway at YVR, went to the farmers market and bought some gourmet items, explored more of Granville Island, played on the beach at Kitsilano, walked the docks at the maritime museum, and played laser tag with a family from the house. We also saw 'The Hunger Games' and Jasper saw 'Mirror Mirror' with his friend. Jasper has been teaching himself

"C", a computer programming language, and made a program to tell your Chinese Horoscope. Stephen and I have been working plans up to launch a sailing school endeavor with *Carlotta* and have an engine installed. We are so appreciating the support from all our friends and family and feel like we can see light at the end of the tunnel. - Barb

Sunday, April 15, 2012 at 9:55pm

Jasper got out of the hospital today. So that marks the end of chemo cycle number five. We're all a bit tired but generally in good spirits.

CHAPTER FIFTEEN

THE CHEMO CIRCUS

The children and teen's oncology ward is an amazing place. It can be a place of joy, with the simple smile or laugh of a patient bringing lightness to the mood of an entire room. Also, it can be a place of despair, seeing such innocent lives condemned to such harsh treatments.

The kids are so strong. Many are up against enormously stacked odds. A lot of them are robbed of their futures far too soon. Somehow they find the power and spirit to deal with it. It should be mandatory for adults with cancer to pay a visit to a pediatric oncology ward. Some of them could learn a lot from the strength, resiliency, and courage of these kids. They know how to live in the present, which includes the ability to play and experience joy despite their situation. So even though they're fighting a disease, they are still playing Legos, or coloring artwork, or enjoying a video game. Don't be fooled, a lot of these kids know they are deathly ill, but they choose to keep living in the meantime. They're facing incredible odds and they keep going. They keep fighting. They really are Superheroes.

A lot of the super powers that these kids display are derived from their parents. Being a parent of a child fighting cancer must be *the* single-most hardest role on earth. You can recognize these parents in the hospital – in the cafeterias or waiting rooms. They have sunken eyes of steel from lack of sleep and from having to carry such a heavy load. Sometimes they look like they've been wearing the same clothes for a while. Maybe their hair is scruffy. They carry an air of experience about them – like they know where they are but they've been here for too long. You share a bond with them. When you meet them nothing needs to be said. Sometimes there's a simple head nod to each other while passing in a hallway. Other times you commiserate during the hours spent stuck in yet another waiting room for yet another procedure. Perhaps they are just there for the day for a top up on blood or a check up before going home again. You might see them again in a couple hours during dinner at the Ronald McDonald House where you share a table, or they might be going into isolation and you won't see them again for two weeks.

There are patterns in the day that we all share. We rush so hard to get to an appointment. Then we wait for an eternity. How much longer until the chemo is ready? How much longer until the results come back? Then we rush again to get the hell out of there. We're under pressure all day long – all night long. We've given up our jobs, lifestyle, personal health and hygiene. We've sacrificed our finances. Some have to additionally juggle the needs of other children in their family. It's a huge strain, and sometimes it can irreparably tear a family apart.

It's quite evident just how important the role of a parent is when you see a child without one present. A young teenage boy appeared one night in a room next to ours on the ward. He had a badly broken leg. He had been travelling alone between the homes of his estranged parents when the accident occurred. As a result, he had managed to end up in the hospital alone for the night. I could tell right off he was nervous and scared. He needed some company. I went out and smuggled in a milkshake and burger for him. That cheered him up a bit. All he needed was someone to show they cared - someone to be there.

Sick kids need someone to hold them up, to tell them it'll all be ok, and just to love them. Thing is, so do the parents - but they're forced to just take it and keep going. Every superhero needs a mentor – Batman had Alfred as his father figure. Spiderman had Aunt May to care for him, and Superman wouldn't have made it without the love of Ma and Pa Kent.

> Thursday, April 19, 2012 at 4:07pm
>> The actual 'Bat-mobile' came by the hospital today for tours! Jasper and Noah got their photos taken with it.

Wednesday, May 2, 2012 at 7:42am

Jasper will be on Global TV and CTV today to promote McHappy Day and the building of a new Ronald McDonald House in BC.

Wednesday, May 2, 2012 at 1:23pm

I tanked gas today. You know you're distracted when you try to repeatedly hang up the pump nozzle into the credit card slot...

Thursday, May 3, 2012 at 12:26pm

Jasper got an injection of a new drug that helps stimulate his blood counts. It worked, so today and tomorrow he's hooked up for a stem cell collection.

Thursday, May 3, 2012 at 1:30pm

An update from Barb: We are having an eventful week so I thought it was time to let everyone know how we've been doing. Jasper weathered his recent chemotherapy (April 12-14) like a trooper. He was out of hospital in record time, and more importantly, he has come through the risk period for infections without any hospitalizations! This is such a relief. His immune system is on its way up and he looks well and hasn't lost weight. He is still needing transfusions of platelets and red blood every few days - but this should improve over the next week. Both Stephen and I have had a chance to get away for some time to ourselves. I spent a few days in Calgary helping out my Mom who had been in a car accident (she is fine now - but was very bruised and sore). Stephen had to leave the Ronald McDonald House because he had a cold sore, and spent several days in Powell River reconnecting with friends and spring-cleaning on *Carlotta*. Jasper's case was presented to the Tumor Board a couple of weeks ago, and so we have a tentative plan for the completion of his treatment. He had an MRI on Monday which shows that the cancer has not spread anywhere (i.e. brain or spine) and that there is a small amount of tumor material left in the brain which is likely dead tissue. The neurosurgeon is still examining the MRI to see if he can safely do a surgery to remove it. After surgery, Jasper would have one last round of chemo. Surgery would be late May, chemo in June and hopefully home by early July. If they elect not to do the surgery, he will instead have one last round of chemo...and then focused radiation at the tumor site. We would have a break at home of about a month between the recovery from the last chemo (end of June) and the start of radiation treatments (August) - which would take about four to six weeks. We accept both of these plans although each carries different risks and it is hard to change paths - you do all your worrying over again! We certainly still feel that Jasper is getting excellent care. Many experts are chiming in again from around the world to help determine the best plan. In the meantime, while we wait for the surgery decision, Jasper is back in stem cell harvest mode - which means stimulant drugs and some overnight stays at the hospital: last night, and possibly tonight and tomorrow night. It worked for platelets...so everyone think and pray stem cells! They want to get a back up supply to add to what they have already collected just in case the last chemo treatment takes too hard a toll. Jasper got to participate in McHappy Day by visiting McDonald's restaurants in company with Ronald McDonald himself, and got a quick interview on the evening news from the CTV weatherman! He did great and had an awesome time. In the meantime he has been busy with Lego and computer games and creating his own worlds and creatures on paper and with his computer. He wrote and recorded his own song using his iPad and iRig microphone with GarageBand. We had a mini spring carnival at Ronald McDonald House, and got to spend some time at the school field nearby on Sunday to toss a ball around! It's been a long time since we could play like that - good to see the energy returning! - Barb

Friday, May 4, 2012 at 10:07am

Yesterday we met with Doctors and Surgeons. Jasper will have surgery to remove the remains of the tumor. This will happen in approximately two weeks - or when his counts are recovered from chemo. It's a minimum four-hour operation - probably eight hours long. There are possible short and long-term side effects related to field of vision, eye movement, hearing, etc. The surgeon feels he can safely remove the mass. This will be followed by a consolidation round of chemo and stem cell transplant. Please pray for my son. Onwards we go...

Sunday, May 6, 2012 at 10:21pm

We have taken advantage of a small window of opportunity and have retreated to Long Beach for two days. Jasper is flying his kite and paper model airplanes here. It's been really therapeutic for us all to get away before the next 'shamozzle' of treatment.

Wednesday, May 9, 2012 at 7:50pm

Update from Barb: Just a quick addendum to say that the final recommendation from the neurosurgeon was to go ahead and remove what is left of the tumor surgically. The operation will be scheduled for when Jasper has fully recovered his white blood cells and platelets so that bleeding and infection will be minimized. We expect that will be Monday or Tuesday next week. The surgery is the same as was described to us back in November - fairly involved with a small chance of eye movement loss and peripheral vision damage, although the tumor has shrunk away from the area that involved hearing and music - so losing that is no longer a risk. As the tumor is smaller and less involved due to the success of chemotherapy, the whole thing is a lot less risky and won't take as long as it would have six months ago - but it is still brain surgery and so we are all nervous and it's taking a long time to get used to the idea. Jasper will spend about four days in hospital afterwards, and then will have about ten more days to recover before they start the last round of chemotherapy (Yay!). If all goes well - no radiation is planned. Jasper is feeling pretty well right now. We were able to harvest a few more stem cells last week as a 'back up' but it was hard to be in the hospital for two days when you are feeling good and the weather is nice. When not hooked up to the harvester, lots of basketball and air hockey were played. Zach visited, and once discharged, we were all able to take in and thoroughly enjoy 'The Avengers' on Saturday. We then escaped Vancouver for a couple of days with our friend Chad and we all went to Long Beach, Qualicum Beach to visit Grandma, and Duncan to visit the Timmermans for a smokie roast. It was back to the clinic yesterday - tired and needing blood, and then out to a special night at the Aquarium for all the kids with special challenges. It was great fun. My parents will come out to visit towards the end of this week. Please keep us in your thoughts and prayers. We're almost there, but the hardest parts seem just ahead. - Barb

Monday, May 14, 2012 at 8:14am

Jasper and Opa admired a brand new BMW motorcycle on display at the 'Balding For Dollars' charity event. Might there be a motorcycle in Jasper's future?

Monday, May 14, 2012 at 8:38pm

Today Jasper's counts were very good (bone marrow recovering nicely!) - but not quite good enough to have a surgery tomorrow. It turns out our neurosurgeon mostly operates on Tuesdays - so we are likely delayed until next Tuesday. On Thursday we have an appointment to check counts again and have a preparatory meeting and check up with the anesthesiology team. Then we will be able to enjoy the long weekend, as Jasper is feeling very well.

Monday, May 21, 2012 at 8:41am

We have *Carlotta* in Sidney now so an engine can be installed. Yesterday we all went sailing in the 'Old Gaffers Race' here. It was Jasper's first time on board since he was diagnosed in November and our first sail this year. He's feeling really good and is in great spirits. His surgery is scheduled for May 29th. He says he's ready for it. We have a clinic appointment tomorrow so we will be back in Vancouver for that. All is well. Onwards we go...

Saturday, May 26, 2012 at 8:57pm

This coming Tuesday is Jasper's surgery. We needed a break so we left town on a road trip and drove south to Portland, out to Seaside, and back up through Port Townsend and Whidbey Island. It was a great distraction from the upcoming week. Jasper and Grandma walked together on Cannon Beach.

CHAPTER SIXTEEN

A MIRACLE

Monday, May 28, 2012 at 7:21pm

A miracle. Jasper had an MRI scan late this afternoon to help map the surgery tomorrow. The MRI shows the tumor and scar tissue is five percent the size it originally was. It is the same size as the blood vessels around it! Kind of risky to go after something so small which could all be scar tissue anyways - so no surgery! We are down to a single round of chemotherapy!

Monday, May 28, 2012 at 9:28pm

More details from Barb: Today we had a busy day prepping for surgery - which concluded with an MRI. The last MRI was April 30th so they wanted a more recent one to use during surgery. We were not really expecting any changes and weren't nervous about the MRI like we usually are. We figured it was just a formality. We left the hospital around five o'clock and when we got back to Ronald McDonald House, our neurosurgeon and oncologist phoned to tell us that there had been further shrinkage of the tumor material. The neurosurgeon estimated that there had been two to three millimeters more shrinkage since April, and that there is a strong likelihood that the remaining material is just scar tissue. He said that what is left is about the same size as the blood vessels in that area of the brain, about five percent of the size of the original tumor. Basically the reason for the call was that both doctors had a gut feeling that the benefits of the surgery no longer outweigh the risks. They advised that we not go through with it and after some discussion we agreed. So no brain surgery tomorrow.... if ever! This is a huge relief to all of us as it has been very stressful anticipating this surgery and we are all exhausted. It is taking some time for us to really process it - talk about an emotional roller coaster. We have simply chosen to believe that this is the miracle we have all been praying for. This latest tumor reduction has happened since the last MRI and in that time there hasn't been any chemotherapy! This is the second time that a last-minute decision has been made to avoid surgery - obviously Jasper is just not meant to go through that. The plan to reduce with chemo to the point where surgery isn't necessary has been very successful. We now proceed directly to the final round of chemotherapy - we have an appointment tomorrow at ten o'clock to meet and discuss the schedule. Jasper has to have his hearing and kidney function tested, an echocardiogram, and a dental visit before we start. The oncologist is hopeful that after this round, there will be no cancerous tissue left in the brain. If there is, radiation is still our best option to eliminate it - but less radiation because it is now so tiny. - Barb

Tuesday, May 29, 2012 at 12:43pm

We are back in clinic for some fluids today. Everything is cool.

Thursday, June 7, 2012 at 6:33pm

Jasper's on CBC Television for the groundbreaking ceremony of the new Ronald McDonald House in BC!

Saturday, June 9, 2012 at 6:59am

Jasper has a surgery this morning at eight o'clock to remove the troublesome CVC port in his chest. It has a tendency to clot up and has also been a frequent source of pain in his shoulder where it loops around before going into his carotid artery. They will switch it out with a smaller less troublesome model. It's a simple surgery that takes about half an hour whilst he is under anesthetic.

Saturday, June 16, 2012 at 4:51pm

Three more hours and Jasper is finished with chemo - forever.

Saturday, June 16, 2012 at 6:33pm

Tuesday Jasper goes into isolation. This will be for at least one month. There are strict measures to adhere to during isolation. He will have a stem cell transplant this week. Pray that he can hold off any infections along the course of treatment. He's currently really drugged-up and feeling completely horrible. And he looks terrible. One of the chemo drugs he's on requires he bathes four times a day with a complete change of sheets and pajamas, as the chemical leaches out of his skin. It's a rough time for the brave and strong boy. Barb and I are both tired and stressed.

Sunday, June 17, 2012 at 5:30pm

"If you are going through hell, keep going." - Winston Churchill

Tuesday, June 19, 2012 at 12:51pm

Twin towers of intravenous pumps now.

Saturday, June 23, 2012 at 9:07am

He's not doing so great. He can't keep oral meds down and he's doped up on morphine. Fever. Zero sleep last night. Threw up his NG food tube yesterday.

Saturday, June 23, 2012 at 6:19pm

The NG tube is back in so medications are being piped into him now. The fever has gone down and he is sleeping again. Medications for the cramps are helping now too.

Saturday, June 23, 2012 at 9:11pm

Good night Jasper.

Friday, June 29, 2012 at 8:54pm

Update from Barb: Well - we've been down the proverbial rabbit hole for the past few weeks, and can finally see our way out so I have time for an update. Since I sent out the link to Jasper's appearance at the Ronald McDonald House groundbreaking we've been busy. Jasper had a week's worth of tests to ensure his baseline health indicators prior to this chemo round. This included heart, kidneys, ears, eyes, teeth, lungs, and blood levels as well as meetings with the transplant coordinator and psychologist. All these tests showed him to be in very good health. On June ninth Jasper had a small surgery to remove his centerline, which was acting up, to replace it with a smaller, lighter version that will suffice until the end of treatment. He weathered the surgery well and that evening we escaped to Sidney for a last out-of-town jaunt before the long hospital stay. Stephen was there working on *Carlotta* and we had a good birthday weekend celebration for Jasper; playing games, shopping with birthday money in Victoria and attending Food Fest at Fort Rodd Hill. Jasper was admitted for six days of heavy chemo on Monday June 11th. Two of the chemo drugs were ones he was familiar with, but the third was new, and the key ingredient for this final round, which is intended to mop up any stray cancer cells that may be remaining. This very toxic drug required Jasper to bathe four times daily so that it wouldn't stain and burn his skin! No small feat when you are feeling terrible and attached to an i-v pole. We then had two rest days before entering isolation. One of these was truly a bed-rest day and also saw the insertion of an NG tube (in through the nose, down the throat into the stomach) - which was very difficult and proved uncomfortable for a good week, causing retching and vomiting. The second rest day we managed a short trip to Chapters to stock up on books to read while isolated. To enter isolation everything had to be wiped down with disinfectant, laundry had special protocols, hand-washing for a full minute is necessary every time the room is entered, bedding and pajamas are to be changed daily, as well as daily baths. No library books allowed, and many foods are forbidden (not that it has mattered because he hasn't eaten anything by mouth since we got in the room). Anything that falls on the floor gets kicked out the door. Some restrictions to protect the immune system will apply for six months following the transplant. This round of chemo basically entirely wipes out the bone marrow. Normally this would be a big problem as you can't survive without an immune system for very long, but that's where those stem cells we harvested back in February come into play. They 'rescue' the bone marrow - find their way there and start producing blood cells again. The obliteration is so complete that Jasper will need to repeat all his childhood vaccinations. The stem cells were infused on June 19th - kind of anticlimactic, very similar to a blood transfusion. The only notable part was that the preservative they are in smells like oysters - so the room smells for about 24 hours. Then it's just a waiting game... The day after transplant it was discovered that Jasper had c.difficile - most likely just resident in his own bowel but out of control due to the suppressed immunity. Brutal - lots of trips to the loo at all hours of day and night, and cramping severe enough to require heavy morphine. I haven't been that sleep deprived since he was a newborn! This went on for a good 5-6 days - but we seem to be past it now. Pain meds have been pulled back and Jasper is feeling much better. During this time he got his nutrition by intravenous as his guts were in too much turmoil to accept even the liquid feed through the NG tube - although medications went through there. They told us that it would take between nine and fourteen days for his stem cells to "engraft" and start producing white blood cells again - and sure enough on day nine (yesterday) they started to appear! A huge relief and now it's just a matter of getting to the point where Jasper can take food and drink by mouth again and be finished his course of antibiotics to fight the c.difficile. Once these things are achieved, we may leave the hospital and live at the Ronald McDonald House until Jasper is no longer dependent on transfusions of red blood cells and platelets - which usually takes ten days to two weeks. Sometime in that period I will return to Powell River and the guys will follow when Jasper is ready. It is a big relief to be through the last chemo and on the recovery side of the cycle. So many things could have gone wrong last week that didn't - and even though it was very hard, we are now all relieved and grateful. Jasper has been a real soldier through this most difficult part of his treatment. He has read tons and watched a lot of Star Trek and Big Bang Theory. We have had a few visitors also. He had his birthday in the hospital - thanks to everyone who sent cards and gifts - the hospital staff was also very good to him. Tomorrow they might disinfect the 'playroom' for him and he can spend some time playing air hockey and video games. We will be switching shifts - Stephen will come and spend a few days here and I will go to Sidney for a few days break to play with Pippa and stay with Chad. Almost there... - Barb

Saturday, June 30, 2012 at 8:18pm

Jasper is feeling much better tonight!

Sunday, July 1, 2012 at 1:07pm

A step-down in isolation meant Jasper could leave his room and go outside today.

Saturday, July 7, 2012 at 9:05pm

Jasper's bloodcounts continue to hold steady or climb. He just finished watching a week's worth of Star Wars movies - so he now has an unusually high Metachlorian count too!

Sunday, July 8, 2012 at 4:03pm

Jailbreak! Jasper sheds his prison issue striped pajamas, and his i-v pole from hell, for a two hour pass out of the hospital!

Wednesday, July 11, 2012 at 7:05am

Doctor's say if Jasper continues to improve he may be able to leave Vancouver next week! He is really looking forward to going home. Getting stronger. Won't be long now! Onwards we go...

Wednesday, July 11, 2012 at 8:56pm

Hooray for less gear hanging on the i-v pole!

Thursday, July 12, 2012 at 10:26pm

Jasper is getting discharged from the hospital tomorrow! He has a blood test Monday at the oncology clinic. If all goes well he gets to leave Vancouver that day!

Friday, July 13, 2012 at 12:28pm

Jasper just dragged his i-v pole to the bathroom to pee... only to remember afterwards that he's not connected to it! We laughed.

Monday, July 16, 2012 at 1:00pm

FREE! Free of the hospital and leaving right now.

Friday, July 20, 2012 at 10:31am

Jasper comes home to Powell River tonight!

Friday, July 20, 2012 at 8:51pm

Jasper's home!

CHAPTER SEVENTEEN

WELCOME HOME

Jasper had been so brave and strong in the hospital. I would often be able to diffuse some of the tougher situations with humor. Laughter: it would bring his heart back on the road. Other times, he just wasn't in the mood for it. I'd get the message and back off. Another way to bring lightness to our situation was our at-times blatant disregard to rules in the hospital. The two of us could get up to all manner of troublemaking. It was all harmless stuff of course. Things like pirating the little-blue-kiddy-wagons from the second floor play zone and using them as drag racing carts on the second floor pedway. It was fun to break a few rules. It was our way of saying "Hey - hospital! You can't tell *us* what to do. Take *that*!"

We had terrific support from friends in our hometown. Although Jasper's treatments in hospital were largely covered under health care, there were many additional expenses that we were to face. The community of Powell

River rallied with an ice-skating event at the town's arena, dedicated to raising funds for Jasper, and *Jamming for Jasper*, an evening of musical performances with a silent auction arranged at his high school. We were so grateful for people who sent us donations, and Barb was given the assurance that her job was secure for when she was ready to return to work, plus she was able to maintain her salary on a sick leave. Our small town had a big heart.

A couple of times we were able to fly home to Powell River. A local airline donated several flights to us. Flying home meant a quick twenty minutes in the air. Driving home could be a five to eight hour marathon involving two ferry connections with a long winding road between them. Curled up on the back seat of a tiny compact car for that period of time was not the most comfortable proposition for a cancer patient. We traded this little car for a vehicle he could comfortably travel back and forth in.

We were contacted by the organization 'Make a Wish'. Jasper had earned a wish, so he started making plans for a visit to Japan. Ultimately the destination was changed to Hawaii, as his medical team wanted him in a closer proximity of care, should he require it. Forming future plans like this was important. As a family we tried to still live a life with plans and dreams - to not let our fate be dictated by our current dilemma. We made plans for sailing *Carlotta* and we schemed of future road trips into the US. But it was so hard to think of a future when we were continually dragged back into the hospital.

When we were able to come home to Powell River, Jasper's immune system was perpetually compromised. We were to keep anyone who currently or had recently had a cold or flu away from him. He needed to be in a super clean environment. We all had to religiously practice vigorous hand washing with antibacterial solutions. The regular maintenance and care of the port in his chest also required a sterile environment. Unfortunately, living on *Carlotta* was out of the question. *Carlotta* wasn't easy to access. It was too long of a walk down the docks, followed by lifting oneself up and over the railing to the deck before descending the steep companionway steps. It was just too far out of the limits of endurance of a cancer patient. *Carlotta's* interior was comfortable, but we had decided on a minimalist lifestyle aboard with as few systems as possible. That meant no flushable toilet – instead she had a small portable toilet. There was no shower aboard – we would shower at the marina facilities when required. In fact, the only hot water on board was provided by boiling a kettle. We were all quite willing to live without these creature comforts when we first moved aboard her a year ago, but our circumstances were entirely different now. We needed somewhere we could return home and the heat would be on – not struggling to build a fire in a woodstove and waiting for the hours to pass before the chill came off. He needed a bed, not a bunk that he would have to hoist himself up into. Due to his immune system requirements he was not permitted to drink tanked water either – it had to be from a treated city source. This ruled out *Carlotta's* water tanks, even though they were brand new. All of these concerns added up to *Carlotta* not being a safe or comfortable place for Jasper recovering from his treatments. So we moved our personal effects off of *Carlotta* and rented a house from friends in Powell River. It was located on a hill directly above the marina, and *Carlotta's* topmast with its distinguished burgee was just visible to us from the living room window.

Tuesday, August 14, 2012 at 10:04am

Good news! Today we are in Vancouver for Jasper's check-up - and his MRI scan shows no changes since his last scan. Next week he can have the surgery to remove the port in his chest too. He'll be back in Powell River tonight.

Tuesday, August 14, 2012 at 1:48pm

An update from Barb: So - very good news today! Jasper had his MRI yesterday and it shows that there are no changes since the last MRI on May 31. This means there is a little bit of tissue still in there, but everyone is supposing that it must be scar tissue and that's why it hasn't grown or shrunk. Our oncologist is consulting with a couple of experts at Harvard and Sloan Kettering and our retinoblastoma specialist here at BCCH - one has responded and we are waiting for the others. Generally the options are: biopsy the remaining tissue (which has the same risks as the brain surgery and a high possibility of inconclusive results); treat the area with radiation; or, leave it alone and watch it carefully for the next little while. So far everyone is recommending the last option. Instead of the usual three-month wait until the next MRI, we will only wait two months and check again. In the meantime, no radiation treatment is planned and Jasper will have a surgery to remove his center line (likely next week). By the time the next MRI happens, we should have an opinion from a few more experts. This is an excellent result for Jasper. It was such a good feeling to see our oncologist's confidence and relaxed demeanor about this MRI. Jasper has some scar tissue on his retinas from his previous cancer treatment and we are now feeling like this is all that remains in his brain also. Jasper is just finishing up his final kidney function test and then we are on our way back to Powell River. He can start school in the fall and generally do anything he sets his mind to - including growing some hair! Lately his plans have been revolving around circuit board soldering and building his own electronic devices. He is also looking forward to swimming before the summer is totally over and starting his job at the Library again. We have rented a house for the year and are moving in this week. Stephen is in Sidney preparing *Carlotta*, which will be attending a couple of wooden boat shows at the beginning of September, and we will join him for a bit of vacation. In the meantime we look forward to bike rides, lake swims, the Blackberry Festival, beach time, hikes with Pippa, sailing, and generally some hard earned relaxation. The support from all our friends and family continues as we start to transition back to the life we left. We are thankful for the gifts and kind words, the hugs and tears, the cards, the meals and beds, the storing of our boats and bikes and bedding and dog, the 'Welcome

Home!' signs, extra strawberry rhubarb pies, and the jobs that have been held. This year was a great opportunity for us to realize what a community we are part of. Here's to better times ahead. - Barb

Saturday, September 1, 2012 at 3:15pm

Jasper will be on the 6 o'clock CTV News speaking about the Victoria Classic Boat Show!

Monday, October 8, 2012 at 6:34pm

Tomorrow we are back at Children's Hospital for Jasper's latest scheduled check-up. He'll have a bunch of tests - including an MRI that will give us a current status of his brain. I'll post an update tomorrow night.

Tuesday, October 9, 2012 at 1:03pm

X-ray and chest ultrasound reveals what Jasper had previously suspected: there's a short chunk of his center line that wasn't removed. So he will have to have a surgery to get rid of that - don't know when quite yet. MRI is later this afternoon.

Tuesday, October 9, 2012 at 5:54pm

All is well. No change visible on the MRI. We return in eight weeks. Hooray!

Thursday, November 22, 2012 at 9:18am

One year ago today, Jasper, Barb and I each packed one change of clothes, left the boat and the dog with friends, and headed off to B.C. Children's Hospital, not knowing what to expect. Onwards we go...

CHAPTER EIGHTEEN

IT'S RAINING AGAIN

That was a full year episode of our lives. It had been a year of experiencing extreme ends on a scale of emotion. The crush of bad news followed by the ecstatic joy of a miracle. Heaven and Hell. I could be frightened to tears with fear as my son was pulled inside a giant Magnetic Resonance Imaging machine, and then overcome with grace at the sight of a sunbeam passing through the hospital room window to cast itself across his sleeping cheek.

Jasper had endured so much this past year. I would not wish this shit list on anyone. Procedures. Tests. Appointments. Surgery. MRI scans. CAT scans. PET scans. X-rays. Blood Samples. Medications. Fluids. Pills. Chemotherapy. Blood taken out. Needles. Blood returned in. Transfusions. Incisions. Infections. Anesthetic. Quarantines. Stem cells removed. Bandages changed. Nausea. Loss of appetite. Fluids measured going into him. Fluids measured coming out. Solids measured coming out. Sterilize everything. Implant a CVC port into his chest. Shove NG food tubes up his nose and thrust them down his throat. Vomiting. Dry heaving. Bleeding. Bruising. Burning. Soreness. Swelling. Exhaustion. Hair loss. Weight loss. Fatigue. Diarrhea. Constipation. Fevers. Pain. Yeah, you can see why people take up the lament of "Fuck you, Cancer!" I have witnessed things that should not be seen – things that should not happen - to my very own son. Unbelievably, there were more items to add to this list that were yet to come…

Tuesday, December 4, 2012 at 2:53pm

Jasper had an MRI yesterday. The news is not good. Tumor has spread into Jaspers ventricles where the fluid of his brain is and also there are nodes at the top of his spinal cord. He will have another MRI right away on his spine. Radiation of his entire head and spinal cord will begin soon. Needless to say, we are devastated by this news. But the three of us will keep fighting. We are staying at the Ronald McDonald House again. Everything else is up in the air.

Wednesday, December 5, 2012 at 3:11pm

Fasting all day for an MRI makes a guy hungry so we are at 'Dream Sushi' to reload him.

Thursday, December 6, 2012 at 8:57pm

An update from Barb: Jasper had an MRI on December 3, which has shown that the cancer is spreading in the ventricles of his brain and the upper part of the spinal column. We get the results of a second MRI on his entire spine today. This is unexpected to say the least. We thought we were free and clear, and if there was to be new growth it would be at the original tumor site. Although we all know when cancer starts to spread it becomes much harder to fight and win, our oncologist has been very clear with us: fighting and winning is still the goal here so we have a treatment plan as follows. More of the same chemo will not help. The cells that have escaped treatment so far are obviously not affected by the chemo that was already given. So we are going to do cranio-spinal radiation. This is different than what we anticipated - i.e. we thought we might have to give a focused radiation to the pineal gland. The pineal gland site has actually not changed since May so that wouldn't help either. The radiation has to be to Jasper's entire brain and spinal cord. It is actually fortunate that we didn't do that focused radiation, because if we had, we would not be able to do this broader radiation now, and the focused radiation would not have prevented this spread. There might be some low-dose oral chemo to help make the radiation more effective - they are still looking into it, but have assured us there are no real side effects. Jasper will be fitted for a mold of his head and body on Friday to keep him in the same position for the radiation and then we will go home for a week while they make it. Radiation will likely start on December 17th and is a Monday to Friday affair, each appointment about a half an hour long. Jasper might feel a little nauseous, but otherwise will not feel ill. His hair might thin a little but he won't lose it. A weekly blood test to ensure he doesn't need a transfusion and that's it really - no other pokes – and no need for a center line. If his spine is mostly clear - it will be a four-week treatment. If there are any hotspots on his spine - they'll add a two-week boost to those spots. Our oncologist is almost certain this will stop the growth and spread of these tumors. Once radiation treatment is finished, we will go home for six weeks as it continues to work in his body. Then there will be another MRI to see if it has done its trick. The downside is that radiation can have long-term effects, and in Jasper's case, because he is genetically pre-disposed, that means a higher risk of recurrence. So that, for us, is the hardest news to take. We are grateful to be staying at the Ronald McDonald House in Vancouver again. This treatment plan will involve more travel than last time - but we will benefit from the direct support of friends and our dog at home during it. Jasper will continue with school without much difficulty. Christmas is a special time here, and it looks like we might get a couple of days free from treatment to spend it with extended family. Donations are a great way to support us right now, as although Jasper and one parent and the vehicle are covered on the ferry commute, gas and the other parent are not covered. We need all the positive hopeful energy and prayers people can spare. - Barb

Saturday, December 8, 2012 at 9:10am

We are home for a week. Jasper will be selectively attending school as he wishes. Maybe we can get a day up at Mt. Washington to go skiing. We will be back in Vancouver on Monday the 17th for six weeks of radiation. We'll have a room at the Ronald McDonald House, where we will also spend Christmas. And then there's a two-day break for New Year's, which we will use to fly to Calgary to see family there. Onwards we go...

Saturday, December 8, 2012 at 5:34pm

Friends of Jasper come over to help decorate a tree. I've got the fire crackling away in the corner... a virtual fire displayed on the computer monitor.

Tuesday, December 11, 2012 at 1:11pm

Jasper's mask for radiation treatment reminds us of Star Wars' Han Solo in carbonite. It's custom molded to his head. He's fastened to the carbon fiber table (made of this material so they can radiate thru it) so he doesn't move. And he has an actual tattoo now in the middle of his torso. It's for centering him with the mask and table. Radiation starts Monday.

Sunday, December 16, 2012 at 10:38am

I suggested we go burn donuts in the boat. Jasper couldn't figure out why we would light fire to donuts.

Sunday, December 16, 2012 at 5:26pm

This evening Jasper was emergency airlifted from Powell River to BC Children's Hospital. He's had increased pain in his lower back and frequent shooting pain down his legs that leave him numb with pins and needles. They've put him on a boost of steroids (Dexamethasone) to help. Barb's with him and I'm currently driving south to Vancouver with our gear. He's still in good spirits and smiling.

Tuesday, December 18, 2012 at 12:38pm

Rad is done for today. It went really quick. Now we're at the 'Nice Café' on 8th.

Friday, December 21, 2012 at 8:13pm

Home again, home again bippity boo! We're all rockin' out with beer, pizza and the music of 'Metric'.

Saturday, December 22, 2012 at 10:11pm

Jasper hosts a Minecraft party. Austin, Christian, Jasper, Jeremy, and Joe are here on various laptops and computers. Zach and Ethan are present through wireless.

Tuesday, December 25, 2012 at 10:21am

Happy Christmas! At the Ronald McDonald House.

Friday, December 28, 2012 at 11:43am

Another week of radiation therapy finished. "Home, James, and don't spare the horses."

Tuesday, January 1, 2013 at 3:33pm

This was written by Chelsey Whittle – whom we have shared similar experiences with, as she navigates treatment with her beautiful daughter, Lilee-Jean (Lil' bean). I thought it pretty much summed up my year as well: *"Bye 2012. You may have been better than 2011, but the bar was set so low. However, I learned a lot about myself this year (mostly how to be patient and kind when I want to be impetuous and mean). We did have some triumphs this year, and every day is a blessing. But it doesn't negate the fact that 2012 was an overall shit year. 2013, you have the potential to be the best year ever, so please, don't let me down."* At 10 minutes to midnight last night, Jasper pulled a small clump of his hair out. So 2013 is off to a bumpy start... Still we keep up the fight. Onwards we go...

Monday, January 7, 2013 at 3:31pm

In the radiation therapy wing today: "I'm on the - top of the world, looking - down on creation..." is playing over the speakers. You've gotta love the sunny outlook of those Carpenter's....

Monday, January 7, 2013 at 8:26pm

An update from Barb: Our Christmas and New Year's was pretty good considering. I took a break from pretty much everything over the holidays. We had the radiation mask fitted - which was a very interesting experience. It was made of a malleable plastic that was warmed up to become flexible and then form fitted to Jasper's head and shoulders. He gets to keep it after he's done - it's very Spiderman looking. We keep looking for spiders in the radiation chamber...They say it's impossible... but then that's what they always say just before the superhero is formed. They then did a week of calibrating the linear accelerator for his measurements. The linear accelerator looks literally like a giant KitchenAid mixer! While they were calibrating, we were home attempting a semi-normal week. It was a good week - Jasper went to school part-time and to his job and rehearsals, and got a day of skiing in! We also celebrated an early Christmas with Grandma and you might have heard us singing at the grocery store Salvation Army kettle. Jasper is trying to perfect his Burl Ives style. It was also a very scary week because he was getting increasing symptoms of tumor growth at the base of his spine and no treatment is underway yet. In the end some of these symptoms were so concerning to the doctors that they flew him out on an air ambulance the night of Dec 16th. It turned out all was ok...but it was both frightening and a little exciting to arrive in Vancouver this way. Radiation treatments began on the 17th. Jasper is finding the radiation treatments quite tolerable. Every now and then there is a longer appointment where they re-calibrate things, but generally they only take about 10-15 minutes (which is long enough if you ask me - being clamped in a tight mask!). In order to help him through the time, I read to him over the intercom. We have been reading H.G. Wells 'Tales of Time and Space'. It is fascinating to read predictions of our own time that were made more than a hundred years ago. Wells got so many things right. We even read a reference to 2013 on New Years Eve day that said this was the year that it would become illegal to have any fire or burning that did not completely consume its own waste (i.e. smoke). The team of radiation therapists at the BC Cancer Agency is just incredible. We get such good treatment there. After treatment, Jasper can feel a little nauseous and unbalanced - the nausea was quite bad the first week - but these effects are dissipating as we go. Unfortunately, he has lost most of his hair again - his friends helped him pull it all out this past weekend. But it will grow back. We were all feeling a little sad about the hair loss as his hair was coming back so full and a little bit curly. But it turns out that the bald look is a familiar one for us and not as bad as we anticipated. It's an excuse to go shopping for some more hats, which is on our list this week. Until recently, really the hardest part has been that we still had to control a lot of the symptoms of tumor growth with medication. One of these is the anti-inflammatory steroid dexamethasone - which is nasty. It has side effects including muscle soreness and wasting, significant mood swings, heartburn, and swelling of the face. All of which Jasper has experienced to some degree - although not as bad as some of the cases we've heard about. It also stimulates the appetite -

which is a welcome side effect - and Jasper is enjoying the up-swings of the mood swings. He is slowly being weaned off of it. The pain and symptoms of the tumors are lessening which means the radiation is likely doing its job. Phew. We had a lovely Christmas at Ronald McDonald House with a whole new crew of friends and Jasper was properly spoiled - they gave our family an 'X-box with Kinect' - so now if you see us jumping around erratically through our living room window, we can't just blame the 'Shiny Pennies' (our delicious local micro-brew). We were also lucky to be able to fly to Calgary for New Years to spend with my family, and Grandma joined us there too. We did the full Dutch gig - Oliebollen, Appleflap and a few games of Shulbok. We especially liked re-connecting with Jasper's young cousins. This past week our good friends from Smithers were in town at the Ronald McDonald House. Noah and Jasper reunited over their mutual love of all things Minecraft, Lego, and Star Wars, and topped it all off with a trip to see The Hobbit. We will have a total of thirty-three radiation treatments, which will take us to the last week of January/first week of February (today we finished number thirteen). Throughout this time, as long as Jasper stays relatively healthy, we can continue to come home on weekends, which we are LOVING. Our home is such a great haven and we are so glad to see Pippa our dog and just veg with friends. Because Jasper's bone marrow is tired from last year's chemo, he has had some early reductions in his platelets (which make your blood clot) and had his third transfusion today. Unfortunately, because he no longer has a center line, this means two pokes every time - one for the blood test and one for the intravenous line. He is being a trooper about it. Platelets only last about three or four days in your blood so we will have to carefully time the transfusions so that he can get one just before leaving for home, and then have the next one as soon as he returns to Vancouver. So far, so good on this front. One of the things we are trying to plan for February is a vacation to a sunny spot. Hawaii is high on the list right now. Friends at home have helped with things like Christmas ornaments, our actual Christmas tree (thanks Anna!), sending uplifting emails about all the praying going on, gift cards for coffee and groceries, taking care of our dog and our garbage and our boat, and having us to dinner. It has been good to come home and be able to totally relax. It is worth spreading around that friends from our sailing and musical communities, with help from lots of others, are setting up a fundraising concert evening/auction. It looks to be very musical and funny. I think they are aiming at February 15th and are meeting now and then to coordinate efforts. If all goes as well as it has been we should be able to attend in person. Today marked the end of vacation and the beginning of school and work. Jasper will be trying to keep up a school schedule for a couple of hours a day and I will try the same with work. All the love and support - it continues to sustain us on this crazy journey that feels like it can't really be OUR life sometimes... Jasper is in great form most of the time - he has a terrific attitude and is embracing all the good times and little simple pleasures. We just have to keep our eyes on him if we ever feel discouraged. - Barb

Sunday, January 13, 2013 at 10:15pm

Jasper is working on a project in Jim's shop today.

Monday, January 14, 2013 at 9:42am

To that couple that cut the line at the grocery store: I hope you get sick from those four cans of lasagna you bought. Who buys lasagna at 9am anyways? In fact, I wasn't aware lasagna even came in a can!

Wednesday, January 16, 2013 at 4:08pm

Six more sessions and we are finished with rad therapy.

Thursday, January 17, 2013 at 1:33pm

Geez there's a lot of the patients at the BC Cancer Agency outside smoking. Funny how you don't see that so much with the patients at The Children's Hospital.

Tuesday, January 22, 2013 at 12:03pm

Vancouver General Hospital. One more rad tomorrow.

Wednesday, January 23, 2013 at 10:21am

Last rad therapy treatment today.

Tuesday, January 29, 2013 at 10:57am

Another transfusion today. Red blood cells and platelets - so we are in clinic all day. Blood counts are still trending down so we are in Vancouver for another week again.

Friday, February 1, 2013 at 9:59am

We're starting a platelets transfusion now and waiting for the ANC (absolute neutrophil count) results of Jasper's blood work. A healthy person has an ANC between 2,500 and 6,000. When Jasper's ANC drops below 1,000 it's called neutropenia. Doctors watch the ANC closely because a risk of infection is much higher when the ANC goes below 500. Needless to say, it sets off some alarms when Jasper's ANC drops to 400! So now we wait for the counts to come in, and that'll determine if we get to go home for the weekend.

Tuesday, February 5, 2013 at 11:21am

Jasper has a platelet transfusion this afternoon and then we get to go home! Unfortunately, due to a contagious Norovirus outbreak in Powell River (and Jasper's low counts) the Doctors will not allow us to go to tonight's event – the Concert/Auction for Jasper. And our house will be under quarantine - visitors must be healthy for at least 48 hours prior to a visit. Hand washing is important on visiting too. And not too many people are allowed around him at once.

CHAPTER NINETEEN

PICTURE YOURSELF ON A BATTLEFRONT

Wednesday, February 6, 2013 at 5:57am

Picture yourself on a battlefront. There are bright lights and loud bangs going off around you. People hurriedly scurry past you. Some look you in the eye as they go by, but are only met with your vacant blank stare back. Some shout words of encouragement, telling you that "you're so strong", but you don't feel it. You've seen a lot of action. You've taken a lot of bullets. You were rushed off to this war unexpectedly. There was no warning or tell tale sign of how long you'd be gone for, so you only packed one change of clothes. You look rough. You've been wearing those same clothes for a couple days now. You look tired. You've let some of yourself go a bit. Things like shaving or managing your hair. You've let these things go because all your attention - all your energy - has been directed to the fighting. But this isn't your conventional war of guns and soldiers. This is you and your child fighting Cancer. You're on the front line with him. Heavy aggressive machinery and chemical warfare are pumping into him. Already he's had major surgery to relieve pressure on the brain. A giant scar remains across the top of his head. They've put an access port into his chest. The tubes for it go straight into his heart. You sleep next to him on a cot that breaks your legs and back. You are woken every hour for vital signs. They take his temperature and his blood pressure. They adjust the tubes and wires going into his body. The machines hum all night long, casting their eerie blue and green lights thru your room. All the fluids he consumes are recorded - both coming in and going out. Hardly any food is taken by mouth. The chemo cocktail has tainted the taste buds. Everything tastes of steel. Bowel movements are collected in a white tray. There is pain. God, there is pain. Burning pain. Stabbing pain. Headaches and body aches everywhere. Pills. Always there are pills to be taken. Woken from sleep every night to take them. You are bombarded with medical terminology. MRI scans. PET scans. CAT scans. Fevers. Infections. If it's possible to catch it - he gets it. C-deficile. Diarrhea. Constipation. Vomiting. Dry heaving. He's lost a lot of weight. His skin is pale and paper-thin. His hair falls out. He pulls his eyelashes off. You need to pee? Drag that intravenous stand with you and mind not to pull the tubes out of your chest. 6 months and they've given him as much chemotherapy as he can take. Twice they've come close to killing him. Now they harvest his bone marrow. Hook him up to another machine and completely cycle all the blood from his body three times over. They collect stem cells for a transplant at a later date. For when he "really bottoms out". Blood is constantly taken from his body. Transfusions of platelets and red blood cells seem endless. Blood counts are too low to go out in public. We get a few months of leave from the battle. He grows stronger. His hair grows back. But familiar pains return. The fight is not over. Radiate. Fasten your child to a carbon fiber table. Make him immobile with a tight-fitting mask over his head and shoulders. Close the one-foot thick lead-lined door behind you and then bathe him in radiation at a push of a button. Week after week of radiation. His hair falls out again. His skin burns. And that is where we stand now. The battle goes on. Yeah, we've seen a lot of action. We've seen too much. After spending so much time here it's inevitable that you see death. Death of teenagers, children and babies. That scars you. But how much more can our bodies take? Our minds take? How many more bullets? We are so tired. We haven't given up - but we are tired. Onwards we go...

Wednesday, February 13, 2013 at 1:09pm

Fly in to Vancouver, get some blood, and fly home. Livin' like rock stars.

Tuesday, February 19, 2013 at 7:36am

Jasper's going to school today!

Thursday, February 28, 2013 at 10:33am

Negatives this week: Jasper's had a cold for the past couple days. He's been tired a lot and he has been having pains throughout his body - both side effects of the radiation. Positives: Sunshine peeked through the cloud canopy here this week, my bicycle's wheels spun for an hour, we watched 'Long Way Round' with friends, we've enjoyed eating and cooking, and catching up on lack of sleep. Jasper's been watching episodes of 'V' and 'Terra Nova'.

Sunday, March 3, 2013 at 8:28am

Ski Monday - surf Thursday! Monday and Tuesday we are the guest family at the Ronald McDonald House of BC ski event in Whistler. They have taken care of everything. I get to race in the dual GS (I've pre-packed crutches and bandages), while Barb and Jasper take cooking lessons from a master chef (not a trivial event, as Barb can start a kitchen fire by simply boiling a pot of water). Wednesday morning we will briefly stop in Vancouver and Jasper will have a blood test and checkup before we all travel to Hawaii for some much-needed time away from everything as a family. We come back March 15th for the first MRI since Jasper's radiation treatment ended - it will give us an update on his health.

Monday, March 4, 2013 at 1:51pm

Chilaxin' at Whistler.

Wednesday, March 6, 2013 at 3:59pm

At the San Francisco International Airport.

Thursday, March 7, 2013 at 8:51am

At Kailua Bay. Good morning!

Thursday, March 7, 2013 at 9:38pm

Jasper enjoyed a tasty, colorful shaved ice on the island of Hawaii!

Thursday, March 14, 2013 at 1:05pm

We are back in Vancouver again after a much-deserved break in Hawaii for a week. I am so thankful to everyone who helped make this happen with donations and auctions and such. We were able to escape thinking of hospitals and treatments and instead concentrated on having some fun. Today we are laying low at the Ronald McDonald House. Late tomorrow afternoon is the first MRI since radiation treatment ended - Jasper will be in everyone's thoughts and prayers tomorrow.

Friday, March 15, 2013 at 2:10pm

At BC Children's Hospital having blood work drawn now. The MRI will be between 3 and 5pm.

Friday, March 15, 2013 at 6:09pm

He's still in the MRI machine...

Friday, March 15, 2013 at 7:19pm

Preliminary results look good - the pineal gland has shrunk further. Our oncologist doesn't see anything in the brain and things have shrunk in the spine. She doesn't see any new disease - the radiation is working but it hasn't quite finished its job (it will continue to work for some time yet). However, the radiologist hasn't looked at it yet in detail and won't until Monday when they will call - so we go home tomorrow! More details to come, but for now: dinner. Onwards we go...

Monday, March 18, 2013 at 10:53am

Some good news: The Radiologist looked at Friday's MRI and said, "That looks much better".

Friday, March 22, 2013 at 9:31am

The amount of support in our home community has been truly wonderful. All the financial assistance, and the housecleaning, meals, heating oil for the house, dog watching.... the list is big, and so are the hearts of the people of Powell River. It is greatly appreciated.

Sunday, April 7, 2013 at 8:36pm

Jasper and I went out for an evening stroll together.

CHAPTER TWENTY

DOWNWARDS WE GO?

Monday, May 6, 2013 at 8:34pm

Jasper's been ill all day with some severe headaches, several episodes of vomiting, and numbness to parts of his face. He's been on the couch all day - a lot of it spent on morphine. He seems a bit better this evening now that the headaches have eased. If he's in the same state tomorrow morning they will want him in Vancouver at B.C. Children's Hospital. So - I pray that he gets some rest and healing tonight so he can stay home.

Tuesday, May 7, 2013 at 11:40am

It was a rough night, but today the headache is much milder. He still has loss of sensitivity on one side of his head and he still can't hold anything down. So we're trying our best to hydrate him while we wait to hear back from the team at the Children's Hospital.

Tuesday, May 7, 2013 at 2:16pm

The intense headaches are back. We fly to Vancouver this afternoon for an MRI scan tomorrow.

Wednesday, May 8, 2013 at 3:31pm

The MRI is finished but we won't see results until around 6:30pm.

Thursday, May 9, 2013 at 7:39am

Unfortunately, yesterday's MRI scan shows the cancer has spread extensively through Jasper's brain. Thus we now move from a course of curative treatment to a plan of maintaining a high quality of life for as long as possible. And now these three remain: faith, hope and love. But the greatest of these is love. 1 Corinthians 13:13

Thursday, May 9, 2013 at 11:38am

Almost forgot: Onwards we go...

Tuesday, May 14, 2013 at 4:28am

An update of where we are at... We are in Vancouver for the next few days. Yesterday Jasper started chemo again - a protocol of two drugs taken orally for a five day cycle followed by twenty days off (at home), then repeated. We are now looking at prolonging life rather than an actual cure. In a best case scenario Jasper may see this Christmas. Jasper won't be attending school anymore, although he may drop by for Jazz Choir - and he's keen to do the Jazz choir trip to Victoria this June. He has a 'bucket list' forming. Everything from throwing pottery, getting a tattoo, to hang-gliding! Also, we've chosen to sell our boat, which was a very hard decision to come to as it is tied so much to all our identities. We just don't have the time or energy that she deserves, and our priorities currently lay elsewhere. We've started looking at purchasing a house in Powell River - one that does not require an eight-year restoration! All three of us have lost a bit of the Mohan 'spark'. We are sad and deflated. We are on a slippery slope. I fear that instead of our usual battle cry of "onwards we go" a more accurate depiction is "downwards we go".

CHAPTER TWENTY-ONE

THE DAYS ARE JUST PACKED

Tuesday, May 14, 2013 at 12:48pm

Jasper is testing out trombones at a music store.

Wednesday, May 15, 2013 at 9:19am

Hang-gliding is booked for tomorrow... "We're going out, Marge! If we don't come back, avenge our deaths!" - Homer Simpson

Wednesday, May 15, 2013 at 8:32pm

Today Jasper and I took a new BMW F800 GS motorcycle out for a test ride. Fun!

Wednesday, May 15, 2013 at 9:09pm

We are at a pet store in Richmond, looking into starting a tropical fish aquarium. We jokingly plan a jailbreak for some fish into the Richmond sewer system.

Thursday, May 16, 2013 at 6:27pm

The last couple days have been just packed! Jasper has test-ridden new motorcycles, taken up the trombone, gone to the movies, shopped at Ikea for a new bedroom, released tropical fish into the Richmond sewer system (just kidding), and flown a hang glider in Hope, B.C. He assisted the hang gliding instructor with some technical computer issues at the airport too. I'm unclear whether this computer was just for the hang gliding school, or was actually running the entire Hope airport. We are driving home to Powell River this evening.

Friday, May 17, 2013 at 10:08pm

Tonight Jasper decided to join the cast for the second half of his school's musical "Oliver".

Thursday, May 23, 2013 at 8:13am

Yesterday I made the mistake of looking at a calendar for the rest of the year. Seven concise months laid-out in neat squares. I thought of the song 'Calendar Girl' by The Stars.

Friday, May 24, 2013 at 12:55pm

I fell down today. Physically, I fell onto one knee and rolled onto my side. As I lay there I could feel every odd shaped pebble of the parking lot beneath me press into my arms. I felt empty inside, like I had been 'raked out'. On the outside was the sensation of goose bumps. I fell mentally today. My spirits dropped. I beat myself up over how I've treated family, friends and strangers - lashing out at them, telling them to stay away, treating them badly for no apparent reason. It's a fight not to blame everything on myself. It's a fight to remain positive. I've fallen spiritually. Sometime a few months ago I lost Hope. I suppose it's possible to function without it? Hope seems so based in the future - which seems kind of blank to me. I still have my Faith in God - and I feel it is strong. But there's a rebel in me that finds some kind of satisfaction in listening to XTC's "Dear God". I figure I have a right to be angry to God, but I'm not at a point of dismissing Him or ending my relationship with Him. I still need him. After all, He lifted me up off the pavement today...

Friday, June 7, 2013 at 9:09am

We bought a house! Huge thanks to my old friend Robbie Gomme, who was able to lend us a down payment until our boat sells, to Warren and Rachelle for making so much effort to close the deal smoothly, to Jim and Gerrimae for helping us move, and to Monique for renting us her lovely house this past year. This week we are headed to Vancouver for some chemo and to celebrate Jasper's fifteenth birthday, after which we look forward to setting up our new home. Now we just need to sell our boat so we can buy some furniture!

Friday, June 7, 2013 at 10:59am

We have had some family photos taken by a professional photographer today.

Sunday, June 9, 2013 at 5:59pm

We are at Canuck Place Children's Hospice for a couple days on a trial run. Dinner was great - the cookies here are 'The Best'!

Tuesday, June 11, 2013 at 7:05am

Yesterday we had a 'Family Planning' meeting at Canuck Place Children's Hospice. Barb and I were at one end of a couch - a nurse, doctor, and counselor at the other. We were not expecting the meeting to be so intense. The staff were kind and soft-spoken, but it was akin to being lined up in front of a firing squad of questions - some sharper than others. Words such as "do not resuscitate", "death", "pain", and "deteriorate" rang off at us. For some of these pointed questions, Barb was able to jump in and protect me while I gained composure. Other times I shielded her as best I could. Don't get me wrong - these folks are here for our benefit and want to do right - there's just no easy route to it. The last couple days we've seen Jasper slip downhill a bit. A numbness spreads across his body. He tires quickly. He walks crooked and relies on a wheel chair often. He has muscle pain. Yesterday he started the first of his five days of chemo. Today we visit with our oncologist. All three of us have a nagging sense that we will be encouraged to stay here in Vancouver. Jasper hasn't decided that he likes Canuck Place yet - the verdict is still out. Barb and I are comforted that there is a professional care team close at hand. It is a friendly peaceful environment here. But we also feel the strong tug of home. Having care at home in Powell River is another possible option that is being worked on as well. We look forward to the coming week. Jasper's fifteenth birthday is tomorrow. His young cousins from Calgary will be visiting Powell River. He plans a solstice party next week. He has some electronic circuit pieces arriving in the mail. And he gets to set up his new bedroom at the new house. Onwards we go...

Thursday, June 13, 2013 at 10:35am

Jasper's platelets are low so he will get a transfusion this morning - then we're hoping to be homeward bound this afternoon!

Thursday, June 13, 2013 at 9:24pm

He's happy to be in his new home!

Sunday, June 16, 2013 at 8:10am

The best way to start Father's Day: waking up beside my son. Now if I could just get some breakfast in bed happening around here...

Thursday, June 20, 2013 at 5:07pm

Jasper will be interviewed about the upcoming Powell River cardboard 'Box War' on the show "Lets Talk Trash" on Powell River's CJMP radio at 5:30 this evening.

Sunday, June 23, 2013 at 4:28pm

Today's cardboard 'Box War' was a hit (literally)!

Tuesday, June 25, 2013 at 8:56am

Donations have been a great way to support us - whether it's for fulfilling Jasper's 'Life-Goals' list, or to help us keep our heads above water financially.

Sunday, June 30, 2013 at 9:08pm

This evening Jasper and I went for a motorbike ride. Jasper no longer has the use of his legs, but his arms are strong and it felt good to be held tight by him on the back. We stopped at the 'Top O' The Hill' store for drinks and ice cream.

Monday, July 1, 2013 at 2:23am

Manifest of Evil
Cancer, what have you done with my son?
You've stolen his spirit.
You've stolen his smile.
You have taken his dignity
stripped away his joy
drained him of his blood
scarred and burned his skin
tainted his taste
and left him with brittle bones.
You sheared his hair
and robbed him of balance.
You've crippled his legs
broken his spine
crushed his mind
blinded his vision
and left his body with paper-thin skin.
And still you are not finished.
You continue to slowly tear him apart.
You are cruel, dark and heartless.
Cancer, what have you done to my son?

- Stephen Mohan

CHAPTER TWENTY-TWO

ONWARDS HE GOES

On our first introductory trial visit to Canuck Place Children's Hospice, Jasper had not particularly liked the place. Naturally, he wanted to be at home, so Barb and I honored his request to stay in Powell River for his palliative care program. Our new house ticked all the right boxes: level entry, germ and dust free, and stocked with mobility aids and extended care assists.

I could expound a chapter's worth of material on Jasper's current condition – about how bad things got. But I will not share my son's state of ill being here, out of respect for him. I will not share how badly the cancer had taken hold and torn him apart – debilitating his beautiful body and robbing him of his clever mind. He would not want that recalled here. Nor can I bring myself to write it...

Suffice it to know that Jasper's level of pain quickly outgrew our best efforts at managing it. Barb and I became exhausted. We had a standing offer to stay at Canuck Place Children's Hospice if we needed it. We wanted to honor Jasper's wishes to remain at home, but it was evident that his pain was too big for us to manage alone. We left for Vancouver, all three of us in need of the hospice to catch up on rest and pain control.

Tuesday, July 2, 2013 at 3:17pm

We are at the Canuck Place Children's Hospice. We are here for a 'tune up'. Jasper can get up to speed on some pain management and Barb and I will catch up on some much needed rest. Hopefully we are home again in a few days.

Sunday, July 7, 2013 at 3:54pm

Last month, Jasper decided he would like to plant a tree in our front garden. At our local garden center we decided on a Cherry tree, because Jasper wanted something that would bloom with beautiful flowers in the spring. The three of us were all in tears when we realized that Jasper would not live to see another spring of Cherry trees in bloom. We left the garden center filled with sadness - and without the tree. Strolling the gardens today at Canuck Place Children's Hospice I found a plaque with this poem:

A Shropshire Lad II: Loveliest of trees, the cherry now

Loveliest of trees, the cherry now
Is hung with bloom along the bough,
And stands about the woodland ride
Wearing white for Eastertide.
Now, of my threescore years and ten,
Twenty will not come again,
And take from seventy springs a score,
It only leaves me fifty more.
And since to look at things in bloom
Fifty springs are little room,
About the woodlands I will go
To see the cherry hung with snow.

- A. E. Housman

Wednesday, July 10, 2013 at 11:34am

Hope Has Fallen Away

Hope has fallen away. It lies in the muddy ditch by the roadside, trampled by the passing horses and carts. It is mangled and bent and cannot be reformed. But: "There is always Hope". Is there? I can only see one inevitable outcome. The way has been lost. I see it in your sunken hollow eyes and how you struggle to hold your head up. 'The Battle' is lost. It is over.

And yet, 'The Fight' goes on around you.

There is still a light in your eyes - a spark that could ignite a fire. So, something of you is still there. Knock off the heavy burden weighing down on your slouched shoulders. Get up. Keep going. Take up the broken piece of Hope by the side of the road. Force it and stretch it for all you are worth into a shining shield. Gather up your remaining strength and couple it to your Faith with Love. Make your last stand one to be remembered. Hope for one more day. Hope for one more breath. Hope for one last kiss. Live your last breaths on your own terms as you go off in one final dazzling display of white light across the sky.

– Stephen Mohan

CHAPTER TWENTY-THREE

WEIGHTLESS

The room at Canuck Place Children's Hospice is on the second floor. It is a warm July evening. The window is open wide. A gentle soft breeze lazily billows the curtains into the room. There is a strong perfume of flowers being carried in from the garden below. Jasper is sleeping.

Days earlier, we all made the decision for the doctor to administer a heavy sedative to allow Jasper to sleep and give him respite from his pain. Later, we realized that he might not wake again during his final days. Now, even though he sleeps, his body still shows signs of pain. Barb and I allow further sedatives, necessary to quiet these tremors and offer him some relief. I think this is what selfless love looks like: our ability to let Jasper be free of his pain put before our desire for him to remain awake with us.

We push a second bed together against his. The three of us are lying close. I am in the middle. It is peaceful. I am listening to his breath. It is slow and labored. It stops occasionally, and then it begins again with a deep rasp. I watch him. He is so beautiful. Briefly, his body lightly shudders in reaction to the pain it is encountering. I am determined to remain awake and vigilant for all of his final days and nights on this earth. I fight with all I have to stay awake...

I wake up. His breathing has slowed considerably. I must have been subconsciously listening. The three of us have a powerful connection: pure Love. I wake Barb. I tell her softly, "I think he's getting ready to go." Barb reaches across me and places a hand on his chest. She can feel his heart slowing. We kiss him and hold him... and then he's gone.

Free of his suffering. Free of the weight of his body. His Soul free to transition and leave uninhibited through the open window.

JASPER SOLO MOHAN

June 12, 1998 - July 10, 2013
Onwards he goes...

CHAPTER TWENTY-FOUR

HOUSE FULL OF EMPTY ROOMS

It's midday and I'm lying under a quilt on the couch. It starts with a jittering sensation in my torso. I can feel a hollow void inside my core – as if I've been inflated like a balloon, but too far – and without the air. My heart is an uncomfortable drum. I heave my body to roll over with the hope of finding a new position to alleviate my numbing left arm and hip. It's no more comfortable than the last, and I roll back again to where I was. I itch and ache everywhere at the same time. Muscles and limbs sag and slump away from me. My head feels like it's caught in a tight steel trap, with the trap's chains running down the back of my neck into my shoulder blades. There's a ringing thrum of tinnitus echoing through my skull. I press my forehead deeper into the pillow so as to block out all the light. A slideshow of images plays out before my eyes. I see all sorts of pictures of things that are beyond my control. There are flashes of the daily news: of terror in the world. There are shots of torrential rains and horrific windstorms. There are pictures depicting the unbearable pressures of tomorrow, and there are glimpses of Jasper from my past. I beat myself up with thoughts of unfounded regret and remorse. I scold myself for what a mess I have made and become. Then the worry creeps in. What have I got in the fridge for supper? Do I have enough money for paying that bill? What if I...? How can I...? They're seemingly endless questions. Most are trivial worries, but I somehow build the molehills into insurmountable mountains. If I can just get myself to fall asleep again I can escape it all. But if I fall back asleep how will I ever be able to sleep through tonight? The thought of another restless sleepless night is the last worry to pass through my thoughts before I once again drift off...

Jasper's cancer journey took a toll on me in so many forms. Mentally, I was a mess. I had spent too long a period under the weight of stress and responsibility for Jasper's care. I had not slept properly for months at a time during his treatment. And while the antidepressants I had been taking for the past year-and-a-half had been an effective tool for helping me contend with anxiety and panic attacks, I felt they also dulled my senses. They had allowed me to cope, but muddied my ability to process my emotions properly. I was skeptical whether the person I was under the effects of the medication was a true version of myself.

Physically, I had completely let myself go these past two years. In hospital, when an opportunity had provided me a moment to myself, I spent it either catching up on sleep or getting some food in me. There had been a kitchen for patient use on each floor of the hospital, but it was only permitted for the storage and preparation of food for the patients. So if Barb or I needed a quick bite, the option was either the cafeteria or the coffee shop downstairs. Subsequently, drinking coffee had suddenly become habitual. The two hospital food offerings didn't really provide anything close to a healthy meal – it was comfort food. There was however always 'real' food available at the Ronald McDonald House. Charitable groups would often donate their time to cook dinner in the house's kitchen for all the folks staying there. This was always well received and appreciated, but again – it was usually heavy comfort food. Beggars can't be choosers, and I happily filled my plate. I was putting on a fair amount of weight. Exercising wasn't an option – there was zero time or mindfulness for that. Heck, sometimes I was lucky if I had the time or energy to shave or shower. My main priority was Jasper.

I had also developed severe sciatica down my right leg. This was from a combination of the tortured hospital cot I slept on beside Jasper's bed, and from constant slouching or napping in unsupportive chairs. A doctor recommended I visit a chiropractor, but half a dozen appointments did nothing to rectify it. I would continue to lumber on through the pain and discomfort. I reaffirmed to myself that the priority was Jasper. I would take care of my issues later, after we got through all this.

But there was a bigger monster looming now that Jasper had passed away - something that I never saw coming. Now, on top of all these ailments, the element of grief was thrown in. Grief can be a cold-hearted bitch of a creature to wrestle with.

When Barb and I returned home to Powell River alone, the first thing I had to do was rid the house of all the assisted-living equipment. I did not want to see the medical walker, the adjustable hospital bed, the adaptor for the toilet, or the goddamn wheel chair anymore. I could only see pain and suffering in these items. They didn't remind me of the true version of my Jasper. I rounded up the plethora of equipment, piled it in the garage and made a phone call to have it removed. Barb went through all the medications and bandages and sterile swabs and items for maintenance procedures and carefully packaged them for disposal. I would have preferred to throw a match and light up the whole giant pile.

Later that week, Jasper's ashes were ready to be picked up in Vancouver. Barb and I would drive to Jasper National Park and scatter his remains below Athabasca Falls, in the same spot that we baptized him. We took turns letting him free into the icy turbulent water.

I was taken by surprise by a special moment that occurred during this event. I had been wearing a silver cross as a necklace the past year. This crucifix was made of two separate pieces – an outer cross that supported a second smaller cross that fastened inside. When Jasper died, I had attached this smaller cross around his neck. I had not expected it to survive the heat of cremation. I never thought I'd see it again. What an amazing gift for me to feel this distinct solid cross in my hand amongst his ashes. It made me feel that both he and God were present for this event. I now keep that cross as a most treasured possession. It has been reunited and inserted carefully back into the surrounding embrace of the outer cross – wrapping it's arms around the smaller one that was cast through fire.

Barb and I returned to Powell River once again, the empty void of Jasper becoming ever more evident. Thankfully we had Pippa come home to us from the care of our friends. Barb busied herself by returning to work. That autumn we held a 'Celebration of Life' for Jasper at a local church. The very next day was the 'Terry Fox Run', a nation-wide fundraising event for cancer treatment. Many of the friends and family that attended Jasper's Celebration of Life participated in the run that day - including several families we had shared time in treatment with at the Children's Hospital. Jasper would have liked that. He had always been a proud supporter of the event.

I experienced a nosedive that fall. I spent my days hiding inside the house, avoiding going out in public. I slept – a lot, to avoid living. I figured if I was asleep I didn't have to deal with anything. Sleeping was a tool I would use to pass through and avoid entire days at a time. Blinds shut and me under the covers. I felt lost and directionless. Nothing seemed to matter much anymore. I gave up. I would bide my time until someday I died.

But deep inside myself I knew something had to change. Jasper would not have wanted me to be in this state of being. He would want me to live. I needed a plan. I had to get out of the house and fix my broken body and redress my mind.

CHAPTER TWENTY-FIVE

I LIKE TO RIDE MY BICYCLE

My friend Jim invited me along for a trip to the dump. He was clearing a pile of junk from his property and had loaded it in the back of his pickup. I had nothing else going on so I came along for the ride. He backed the truck up to the edge of the unloading area and we stepped out. I think I might have scared him a little when I climbed onto the truck's tailgate and started wildly flailing items skywards, cursing and calling out to whoever was within a half-mile of earshot.

I picked up a large rusted piece of pipe. "*That's* for that rotten doctor that brought those interns into our room at *six a.m.*!" Off it spun end-over-end into the far reaches of the dump.

I chucked a broken toaster oven with far more effort than was required and sent it sailing. "And *that's* for the nurse who treated us like *dirt*!" Jim stood back and let me have at it. When I was done I was left with an immense feeling of satisfaction and release. Jim was simply leaning against the truck with a big smile for me.

Anger – I had a lot of it. And I needed somewhere to throw it.

The first thing I needed to attend to was treatment for my sciatica. A local physiotherapist performed some massages. He also wanted to try a new tool he had just acquired. It was a deep tissue hammer that delivered pulsating electrical punches into the core of my hamstring. It hurt like hell, and I could barely walk after a session, but it appeared to be working.

I had also ended my course of antidepressants. Originally when they were prescribed, the doctor had assured me that they would help me. He told me that ten percent of the population of North America was taking some form of antidepressants, so there was no need for undue concern. I was desperate at the time, so I had not questioned him. It almost seemed too easy. Well, one thing that doctor had never hinted at was just how horrible it is coming off them. I consulted a new family doctor and she advised me on a course of action to wean me off the pills.

Exercise would be my replacement to anti depressants. Barb gave me a birthday present in the form of a voucher for an appointment to see Lorne, an expert fitness consultant, at his own local training facility. Initially, I thought "what a terrible birthday gift", because exercise simply wasn't on my radar yet. Really, Barb was throwing me a lifeline. Lorne and I came up with a plan for routine exercise. We also looked closely at my diet. We determined that I was at least forty pounds overweight. I was the most I had ever weighed in my life. Under Lorne's direction I would follow a low carbohydrate, high fat diet.

Turns out, Barb's birthday present was the ideal gift. I now had a fitness plan and a schedule to work to. Having some direction and purpose for getting up each day was such a positive force for me. I actually enjoyed the challenges of my new diet and it was rewarding to see weekly changes. The fitness training coupled with this new diet was paying off in spades. As long as I kept up the routine, I didn't need to rely on the meds to pull me out of a funk. It was hard work though. Nothing came easy. One of the side effects of the medications I was tapering off of was excessive perspiration during physical activity. Fifteen minutes on the stationary rower or running on the treadmill and I'd be drowning in sweat. Other medication side effects included sudden lightning flashes before my eyes, and my body would sometimes unexpectedly deliver a violent twitch – strong enough to wake me from sleep at night.

I religiously stuck to my new exercise protocol, in conjunction with regular massage and physiotherapy treatments, and careful attention to my diet. My sciatica was subsiding. The excessive weight was shedding fast too. This became evident when I decided to add some lane swimming to my routine. I had not swum lanes for years, but I figured "Hey, it's like riding a bike, you don't loose your swim skills." On my first visit to the pool I performed a shallow entry dive. "Yeah", I thought confidently to myself "I still got it." All elegance of form vanished when I surfaced in the middle of the pool with my trunks around my ankles. Also, my prosthetic eye had dislodged itself from the impact of the dive and was now rattling loose inside my ill-fitting swim goggles. I had lost so much weight in my face that my eye no longer fit properly, and my swim trunks were far too large a size for my now slender frame. I made a hasty retreat to the men's change room.

Bicycles had figured so prominently in my past, it seemed only natural that I would gravitate towards them again. Cycling proved to be a fantastic outlet to channel energy. There were a couple of weekly scheduled group mountain bike rides in Powell River that I started to tag along on. Socially it was good for me to get out and mix with other people again, and everyone I rode with was very supportive of me and keen to keep me riding.

I recall watching video footage of cyclist Lance Armstrong visiting a children's oncology ward. He commented that all the challenges of racing in the Tours, together, are nothing in comparison to what the parents of these kids are going through. I kept this in mind when I dove back into cycling: that I've already come up against the hardest challenge of my life, and therefore anything difficult that cycling presented I could manage and meet with strength and determination.

I took a position once again working part time at Suncoast Cycles. Frank, the owner of the shop, went out of his way to accommodate my needs for a casual position with a flexible schedule. This was important, as being out in the public eye was still pretty raw for me, and my ability to juggle grief with a job was not easy. The job kept me occupied, and it fueled my obsession to ride by providing me with an employee's discount for use toward a supply of bicycles and cycling gear.

The shop was a proud supporter of the 'BC Bike Race', a series of mountain bike races that toured through British Columbia communities each summer. Powell River was part of its circuit and the local cycling club wanted to build a new section of trail to highlight the race. I felt this trail needed something unique that would showcase the area to this international group of racers. I scouted out the newly planned trail and found an opportune spot to build an out of the ordinary overpass bridge. My idea was that riders would climb a narrow gully, passing under a forty foot long arched bridge spanning the gap above them, then they would sweep up and around a large curve to the right, before continuing over that same bridge and thus onwards up the trail. There certainly wasn't anything like it on the race's tour. I could see race day playing out in my head - a long convoy of riders passing under, over and around the bridge all at once. What a remarkable sight that would be.

The club gave their approval and I set to work. It was to be constructed mostly out of materials on site. The majority of the bridge I would end up building alone. I'd be twenty kilometers up a forestry road by myself in the woods, busying myself with the heavy labor of driving big timbers together. This would prove to be good therapy for me. I was immersed in a project, with my mind and body occupied on a task again. I so badly needed a sense of accomplishment. I needed to feel that I was *doing* something.

I started by timber cruising the immediate area for the pair of long arched spans that would give the bridge the unique character I was imagining. Anyone can build a straight bridge with ninety-degree angles and square corners - I was envisioning something special with elegant curves. After a couple of visits, I found a dead tree that would perfectly fit the curved shape I was after. Unfortunately it was still standing, leaning at an angle of about sixty degrees from horizontal. Also, it was snagged, one-hundred-feet up, in the canopy of the several other trees surrounding it. I double-checked it was okay to use the tree with the club. They would bring in a professional faller, since it appeared it was going to be especially tricky to fall this tree. In the end, no one wanted to touch it. It was far too dangerous a feat, and put the chainsaw operator in peril of being crushed.

Well, I had already waited a week for this unwanted news and I was anxious to start, so I figured "What the heck, I'll cut it down myself. *I've got nothing to lose...*"

John Wayne said, "Courage is being scared to death, but saddling up anyway."

I went forth to fall the tree myself. To say there were some tense moments is understating it. I successfully made the saw cut through the trunk and was greeted by the false start of the tree falling. It promptly stopped its descent and was now fifty degrees from horizontal. What I found most alarming was, while the trunk was free from its stump, it now happened to be hovering precariously four-feet off the ground. The rest of the one-hundred-plus feet of tree was still hung up in the surrounding forest above.

John Wayne is also attributed to the saying: "Life is tough, but it's tougher if you're stupid."

I tied one end of a long length of heavy duty, four-inch wide webbed truck strapping as high as I could reach up the trunk. The other end – let's call it the 'stupid end', I attached to a steel hook on a wire rope that lead to a 'come-a-long' ratchet tool. I stoutly anchored this tool with wraps of chain shackled to a nearby tree. I took up position at the stupid end. Here I stood ready to winch the unsupported three-foot diameter base sideways and downward. My heart raced. Again: "What have I got to lose?"

The first pulls on the ratchet proved fruitless. The tree barely budged. I managed to pull a couple more swings on the ratchet's handle. My apparatus of strapping, chain, and wire came under extreme high tension. Clearly I now had all my gear pushed beyond any manufactured limits: if something snapped I would be in the direct line of fire and at risk of serious injury or death. Also, there was no telling what would happen to the gear once the tree started to fall. The trunk could kick out on its descent in a direction that might pull my winch line to its demise. So not only was I at risk of the trunk swinging into me, but also of the winch line breaking and cutting me in half like an enormous steel whip.

I glanced around at my surroundings and planned a quick escape route in my head. I gave one more 'click' to the ratchet and the tree moved slightly. So much tension now... one more click should do it. I pulled the handle and didn't even wait to see the result. Without looking up or back, I sprinted away as fast as I could on my predetermined escape route, crashing my way through the bush. As I ran, the anticipation of something about to crush or cut me in half was heavy on my mind. "Am I safe? Did I get away with it?" Thankfully, my questions were answered by the heavy 'whumph' of the Giant falling to the forest floor behind me. "I did it! *And* I'm alive!"

Now that the tree was finally on the ground I could cut out the forty-foot length I needed and move it to the bridge site. This was about 200 meters away on a slight down-slope. It was heavy, backbreaking work, laboring all by myself with this big, roughly hewn piece. I would use the webbing straps and the come-a-long to shuffle the beam a couple of feet at a time. The problem I now faced was that the beam I had cut was curved like an enormous banana, so every time I got it to start moving under its own inertia, it would skew off in a completely new direction with a mind of its own. It simply refused to take the straight direct path I wanted it to travel. A few times it abruptly stopped by wedging itself between a series of trees in its path, stuck fast with its six hundred pounds of weight behind it. Many times I had to heave it *back up the slope* to get it pointed in the proper direction again. It could take an hour to move it six feet. Or it would somehow find a hare-brained route through the trees and I would cheer its ever-closer progress towards the site. It was an exercise in patience and futility (or 'stupidity', according to John Wayne).

Pippa and I would drive up from town in the morning, light a campfire, and spend the better part of a day on bridge construction. The cycling club held a couple of work parties on the trail, and I was happy to have volunteers assist in skinning the bark off logs, clearing the bridge site of boulders and fallen debris, or lending a strong back to erecting the supporting vertical posts. In the end the bridge turned out to be its own little marvel of engineering deep in the woods. The club named the trail 'Aloha' (for some obscure reason), so I carved the name into the main beam of the bridge. At one point the club asked me if I wanted them to rename the trail 'Jasper's Way', but so many folks already knew the trail under its current moniker that I didn't see a rename in order. Besides that, I had already scribed the Aloha name deep into the bridge spans.

What a treat it was come race day. Just as I had previously imagined, I watched a train of B.C. Bike Racers snake their way under, around and over my bridge. The bonus, when they reached me cheering with my cowbell at the top of the gully, was that they were all smiles.

Following the Aloha bridge construction, I spent some more 'me time' in the bush closer to town building another mountain bike single-track trail. I also dabbled in some mountain bike racing for a season. I enjoyed the competitive aspect, but then it quickly dawned on me that the pressure of racing was creating stress and anxiety, so I backed out at the end of the season.

Some friends in the mountain bike groups were also road cyclists. They suggested I start riding road bikes with them. This was something I had not done since the summer I rode into the trunk of that car, back when I was eighteen. Turns out I had really missed being on a road bike. It was a terrific sport to be a part of again. I loved the feeling of going effortlessly fast, lightly tapping out a rhythm on my pedals and watching the world whiz past. It made me feel free and unencumbered. I could disappear for an entire day on my road bike. I took an interest in riding longer distances, in particular Gran Fondo (Italian for 'Big Ride') events. I especially enjoyed participating in the Gran Fondo from Vancouver to Whistler. The day before the event I rode the 100 km from Powell River into Vancouver. Then the day following the 125 km event I rode back from Whistler to Vancouver again. I was quickly becoming addicted to this new obsession and I was piling on the miles.

Although cycling and exercise were certainly helpful and healthy lifestyle choices, things were still not all rosy. I found that if I went multiple days without exercise I started to tank and slip back into a depressive funk again.

This was often accompanied by anxiety attacks. Also, I was continually plagued by a lack of sleep. A few nights in a row of poor sleeping with a hit of anxiety could trigger a rough cycle that was hard to break out of. My mind would race with all manner of disconcerting dark thoughts.

That reckless 'devil-may-care' attitude I had while cutting down the tree for the Aloha Bridge seemed to prevail and speak to me often. "With Jasper gone, what *have* I got to lose?" Walking on a busy street or riding my bicycle in traffic was a bad time to hear that voice. It would lead to the urge to deliberately drift out in front of a passing bus or truck. Or it would cause me to briefly pause over the sharp kitchen knives in the cutlery drawer while I was putting away the dishes. Sadly, I went off the rails a couple times and decided to give up. Once I went as far as 'erasing' myself before a planned departure from this world. In the period of an afternoon I put all my belongings and personal effects into storage, deleted myself from social media, and hid anything in the house that had any form of association to me; thus erasing any evidence of myself. I was going to 'check out' permanently.

I'm happy to report that (obviously) I did not follow through on any of my suicidal tendencies. During the last incident, I found myself diverted somehow to a coffee shop instead. It was a late Friday afternoon and there were parents and grandparents sitting with children at many of the tables, the children having just been picked up from school. Seeing these families sharing a treat and a hot drink reminded me of how Jasper and I would spend our Friday afternoons in a similar fashion. I like to think Jasper was present that afternoon and steered me clear of harming myself.

It's hard to get back from those episodes though. For one thing, it's super exhausting and taxing on your body and mind afterwards, and it's difficult to reconnect with people again after socially backing yourself down a hole to disappear. They want to know where you went, and then you've got to somehow explain it all... It's not something that's easy to admit or throw into a casual conversation at the grocery store.

"Hi Stephen, how are you? I haven't seen you around."

"Oh, yeah, I'm fine. I was going to throw myself off the cliff up at the gravel pit last week, but I decided not to. How are you?"

I wish I could report that I am cured of these afflictions. I wish I could tell you I sleep right through the night, and that I don't have those dark thoughts. I so want to be rid of the weight of loss that pins me beneath the covers, but grief is something that doesn't have a cure. Grief is complicated. I will live with it the rest of my life. There is, however, hope for some respite from grief. In addition to cycling, I have found some techniques and practices that provide me with coping mechanisms for grief.

Barb and I agreed I should seek some external help. She has always been a massive support for me and I feel I can share anything with her, but I needed some professional help. I looked to counseling for assistance.

Half a dozen counselors and a Psychologist later (the majority of which, oddly enough, all shared the name 'Lisa') and I've learned some techniques to soothe some of the symptoms of grief that plague me. Some work for me, others... not so much. Massage therapy. Reiki. Yoga. Meditation. Remembering to breathe in and out. Prayer. Exercise. Diet. Group therapy. Writing! I've come a long way from hiding inside with the curtains drawn for days on end. And I'm proud of myself for still making an effort to heal and keep going. Patting myself on the back helps too.

Lately, I've had positive results with visits to a specialist using Eye Movement Desensitization and Reprocessing (EMDR), a form of psychotherapy used successfully for people suffering the effects of PTSD. At first I doubted its effectiveness on me. I mean, it's based on eye movement and I only have one eye... All levity aside, it does seem to be helping. Apparently our bodies have no sense of time, so my body still carries the trauma of having an eye removed and the radiation it experienced as a baby. That traumatic response can recur when it's triggered by the familiar sounds and lights of a hospital – such as our time in treatment with Jasper. EMDR has helped me to revisit some of my past experiences and release the trauma that my body has stored in its cells.

One giant strain and source of anxiety for me was *Carlotta*. Despite having rebuilt it from one end to the other, I was still doing constant repairs and upkeep. Going down to the boat to lose myself in work wasn't accomplishing the same effect as working alone up in the woods on mountain bike trails. There was too much evidence of our past life on the boat, and it was impossible to be truly alone on the docks; there was a constant stream of visitors asking questions about *Carlotta*. If I only had a dollar for every 'dockside admiral' that proclaimed: "Now *that's* a labor of love." and then strolled away… (unbeknownst to them, the fellow behind them was preparing to throw a hammer in their direction). Most folks were genuinely interested in the boat and what I was doing with it. Some would probe deeper with their questions. Eventually the questions would lead to me exposing myself and revealing that my son had recently died. This was not always something I was prepared for, and certainly not what they were expecting.

You would think that with *Carlotta* at only fifty-feet long, there must be an end to the work required on her. Nope. A wooden boat of that size and age really benefits from someone living aboard full time and it needs to be in regular use, otherwise it starts to deteriorate quickly. Unfortunately, during our time in treatment *Carlotta* largely sat un-used and without the full attention to maintenance she deserved. The exception was the effort we made to have an engine fitted in her, but that had been an immense strain on us at the time. After that, Jasper started going downhill and I was only able to just keep up on the bare minimum maintenance required, if even that.

We didn't have the financial means to keep living ashore as well as keep the boat. I was tired and lacked the energy to put into her. I found it an effort to even go visit her at the dock to check on her. Most of the caretaking ended up falling to Barb. I just didn't have anything in me for *Carlotta* anymore. Something had to give.

It was a difficult choice when Barb and I had made the decision to sell *Carlotta,* as the boat had really become a part of our family's identity. I hauntingly recall how very upset Jasper was when I told him we were to sell her. To this day it still carries something shameful for me. I feel like I let him down tremendously. All those years we had shared the dream of rebuilding and living aboard and sailing a pilot cutter. He was always so very proud of the boat, to the point that it was often the topic of his artwork or essays at school. He had helped me with projects on *Carlotta* too. He knew all the details of the history of Bristol Channel Pilotage, all the parts of a gaff rigger and everything to do with wooden boat construction. He had made friends through the boat. He had grown up with it around him constantly. It was an important part of him. He was *Carlotta's* biggest fan. Then I dashed it all by the announcement that we were putting her up for sale. In the end we didn't sell the boat until two years after his death, so maybe I carry that guilt for no reason?

Word got around that we were selling her. There were actually some folks in the wooden boat community that jeopardized a couple of potential sales. They couldn't fathom that we would sell the boat after such an incredible effort to rebuild her and thought we were making a big mistake. After Jasper passed, some people thought we could 'overcome' our grief by getting back into the boat again. I know they meant well, but I felt they didn't fully grasp the ordeal we had been through. They missed the point that it was *just a boat*. We had lost our *son*!

In reality, we needed to sell either our house or the boat to repay the money we had borrowed from Robbie. He had been very patient and had gone above and beyond by lending us the money for the house when we so badly needed it for Jasper. But we had never intended the loan to be carried for this length of time. We knew that the boat, being such a unique item, would take some time to sell in its niche market. So in desperation to return Robbie his funds, we put the house up for sale too.

Barb and I were feeling lost and figured we would keep whichever item didn't sell. In the end they both sold. It was hard to say goodbye to *Carlotta*, but I just couldn't imagine living aboard or sailing her again without Jasper.

With the house sold and the boat about to move on to her new owners, Barb and I decided to make a move away from Powell River. Living there for twelve years, we had put down a lot of roots. There was evidence of Jasper everywhere. That was hard to move away from, but also somewhat easier to not see it all the time in our face. It wasn't easy living in such a tightknit community now either. They had always been so supportive of our family – both before and after Jasper's death, but such a small community can be a curse as well as a blessing. For instance, if I was grocery shopping and someone gave me a 'puppy dog eyes' look of concern, it could cause me to fall apart – even though I'd been previously having a *good* day. Barb and I told ourselves that Jasper would have moved away to go to university anyways, and that it was always our plan to move away from Powell River when he did. So we prepared to leave town.

Without the constraints of owning a house, and with *Carlotta* moving on, it seemed like an opportune time to move. We didn't own any furniture, we had sold our vehicle, and all our possessions fit into a one-bedroom apartment. Barb and I looked to new horizons across the Strait of Georgia to Vancouver Island, close enough to return and visit our old friends and community, but far enough to begin something new.

CHAPTER TWENTY-SIX

BREAKING THE CHAINS

It's springtime on Vancouver Island. It's been almost four years since he died. The approach of Easter and the expectant bloom of the cherry trees bring a poignant reminder of the passing of time. I'm hunched over the kitchen table looking at a map of the western USA, planning another motorcycle trip. I have a new BMW Adventure motorcycle. I need to escape. I know a lot of people plan a trip like this to 'find themselves'. I'm looking to lose myself. My finger traces over a highway in Utah and I have a passing thought of the prophecy I had as a teenager – the one where I'm riding over a cliff with my hair on fire. How ridiculous it seemed at the time. I smirk at how plausible an ending that might make now. Nah… it's still ridiculous.

Last year, I put over fifteen thousand kilometers on the odometer of this bike in just three months. Onwards we go. I have to keep moving. Forward. I can't sit still for too long before my mind begins to race with negativity. On that trip, I packed the bare essentials for camping into the saddlebags and made strides southward. I travelled all over the western face of North America. For the first while it was a terrific form of escape for me. I was alone with my thoughts in my helmet, and I was roaming free without a schedule or a plan. If bad weather showed on one horizon, I would turn and head to the other. Folks I met would ask where I was going. "Oh, I dunno. I'm just wingin' it." They liked that answer. Perhaps it was the sense of freedom that came with it. To them I appeared as some kind of unrestricted cowboy roaming the west. Little did they know the heavy weight that I pulled behind me on that bike, and they wouldn't have guessed I was sometimes using it as a tool of self-flagellation. I'd seek out forms of hardship on it. I'd ride it intentionally through a high mountain pass, my arms so cold I could feel stabbing tentacles of pain spasm down through my wrists. I wanted to feel the sting of hot desert sand blowing in my eyes. I needed the uncontrollable shivering in my core that the pelting of freezing rain delivers at a hundred miles an hour. I wanted to take risks – to push my anxiety past its redline. That's why I buried the throttle in a sideways dust storm coming out of the west end of Death Valley – not really caring if I got blown over the road embankment. That's why I camped in remote solitude far off the beaten track. I was letting loss be my guide.

I was searching for something, though I didn't know what, or where it was. On a whim I decided to go on a pilgrimage to the location that U2 photographed its iconic 'The Joshua Tree' album artwork. I'd always been a fan of the album. It had played a lot through my helmet on that trip. Apparently, the actual Joshua tree photographed for the album succumbed to a disease and died in 2000, and a new tree had since grown close to its remains, along with some other items fans of the band have contributed. I spent an afternoon tromping thru the sweltering desert heat in my motorcycle gear looking for a plaque that marked the spot. I had read that the plaque was inscribed with: "Have you found what you're looking for?" I armed myself with directions, photos and instructions and... I didn't find it. At first I was quite disappointed. I beat myself up over it. "Why does everything have to be so hard? What the hell am I doing out here?" Then I had a revelation: maybe I wasn't meant to find it – 'cause what *I'm* looking for is not at that spot. That tree is not there anymore. It's dead. And like that beautiful unique tree that died too soon of disease, perhaps some of the things I'm looking for can't ever be found again either... I figured I was done searching there. I queued the song to play in my motorcycle helmet, cracked open the throttle, and pointed the bike out of the desert toward the mountains. I still hadn't found what I was looking for. Onwards we go.

I truly was 'wingin' it'. I made minimal plans and didn't have any particular destination in mind. I wanted to get lost. I already felt personally lost, so I wanted to glaze it by being physically lost too. Completely surrendering my sense of direction. Let fate play its card. And it worked...

for a couple of months anyways. Sure, it's great to have all these adventures in foreign lands on a motorbike, and after watching Jasper take his last breaths, I can't help but feel a newfound appreciation for being alive and wanting to experience these grand new adventures; but as time and the miles passed, the effects of escape withered. As Hemingway wrote: "You cannot get away from yourself by moving from one place to another." Something was most definitely missing from the experiences now. Jasper. I felt his void.

As time passes and I get older, I wonder what my odds are as a cancer survivor. Will I live to eighty-three? God only knows. I realize that because of my cancer history that I'm much more susceptible to seeing cancer again. There's an increased risk at this stage in my life that cancer shows up in places like my skin and internal organs - places where cells are still multiplying. With the radiation therapy I had to my head, I'm also at a high risk of cancers occurring there or the brain. Chemotherapy carries added future risk too - higher for those who had it as a child than those receiving it in adulthood. In short: it's a small miracle that I'm still here. That, and the fact I may be sitting on a time bomb.

This means that I need to be vigilant about staying on top of any personal health problems that persist for longer than expected. If I have a particular pain that hangs around I need to get it checked out. That bruise on my ribs – was that from mountain biking last weekend, or…?

I have had a few recent scares that contributed to some sleepless nights. A mysterious lump appeared on my tongue. Luckily that one proved to be benign. But I've also had Basal Cell Carcinoma recurrences around my eyes, which set off some alarms for me. One of these grew quickly to the size of a grape and left me with a three-centimeter scar across my cheek. The anxiety of just being in a hospital again is a lot to bear, let alone lying on a procedure table having your face tugged and stretched while the doctor pulls a disgusting white mass out of your head. Then there's the stress that follows: "We'll just send that off for a biopsy. We'll be in touch." Fortunately, the doctor's do somewhat fast track me through the system due to my history.

One morning, I find myself standing over the kitchen sink, a single pill in one hand, and a glass of water in the other. This is day two of a three-day course of strong antibiotics. By the end of today, this pill should be enough to relieve me of the symptoms of a urinary tract infection. Or at least I hope that's what it is. Oh God, have I got prostate cancer? The two share a lot of the same initial symptoms. Today will determine if I need to go in for further testing. It's a lot for me to process. I become anxious over something as simple as a urinary infection. Of course, my mind plays with the unknown and jumps to conclusions. Any nagging ailment that goes longer than a week moves my personal doomsday clock closer to midnight and the submarine alarm starts sounding: "Aaarruuuugah!"

Fortunately, that night the pain in my nether region subsides. It turns out to be nothing more than a simple bladder infection. It's strange to be happy at that news. "Praise the Lord! I have a bladder infection! Hallelujah!"

Do I *want* to live to eighty-three? It's easy for me to fall into the thought pattern again of: "If I get cancer and die – so be it. I'm ready to move on. What have I got to lose, since I don't have my Jasper anymore?" But I've beaten the odds so well. How can I give up so easily *now*? Especially after being in the company of *so* many children who endured treatment and shared a similar tragic outcome to Jasper. I've come to realize just how much of a special minority case *I* am. I am the living proof that there is hope for a child afflicted with cancer - to live not only a normal life, but an exceptional one. I can't throw that away. Not after seeing so many kids fight so hard to be in this world. I saw firsthand the hell that children go through in the oncology ward – they fight so hard to win. Why do they die and I survive? I've been blessed in that way. I'm the living proof that a childhood plight of cancer can still result in a life lived fully. Parents of kids with cancer need to see that. It would give them hope.

But didn't that hope inconceivably vanish for my Jasper? I'm so conflicted. I'm supposed to be this shining example of survival and a beacon of Hope, but by losing Jasper all I want to do is give up and throw in the towel.

Mom died this winter. It was not a pretty death, if there is such a thing. Her cancer had come back with a slow vengeance. It disabled her across the timespan of a year.

She spent her last months in palliative care, her skin paper thin and blotchy from blood pooling, her body broken from the progression of the disease.

What a different 'end-of-life' scenario it was from Jasper's death. Granted, there are different ways that the dying are going to approach their imminent death, but there was a considerable contrast between Jasper and Mom. Part if it was because of age. Mom was seventy-five. Having cancer later in life is a different proposition. I think this is because you only look forward when you're young. Aged folks are looking back on their life, sometimes with regrets.

At one point the doctors told Mom she might only have a year remaining. She thought it unfair that she should be given this terminal prognosis. Yes, it is unfair for anyone to receive that news, but she seemed to quickly forget how she had abandoned her treatment plan during her previous occurrence. Now she was experiencing the consequences of that earlier decision.

Mom was still totally of sound mind and had her entire mobile capacity, yet she made no plans or dreams to fulfill in her remaining time. She could have travelled the world, or learned to play the banjo, or bought a little red convertible, or moved to a cute little cottage right on the beach, or... Suggestions from Barb and I fell on deaf ears. Instead, she chose to while away the time. She didn't go anywhere. She didn't know what to do with herself, and she made excuses for everything, complaining incessantly. She seemed to give up so easily on so many things. It was frustrating to watch her let go of so much, after witnessing Jasper try to get in as much as he could in his last days. She became rather bitter and malcontent. She did however get blessed with an additional year of life over the doctors' predictions.

In the end, Mom chose to use an assisted death program. She died at her chosen time of 11:30am on a Tuesday in February.

Mom's death drove home a point for me. I need to make a choice: do I choose to live life to the fullest like each day may be my last, like Jasper did, or do I choose to give up altogether, idly passing the hours until an inevitable outcome like my mother? Ultimately: is it better to burn out or fade away?

I choose to burn out. *"Hope for one more day. Hope for one more breath. Hope for one last kiss. Live your last breaths on your own terms as you go off in one final dazzling display of white light across the sky."* I wrote that in my journal just before Jasper died.

This is a hard chapter for me to write. Perhaps it is because of the threat of disappointing the reader. Folks looking for a tidy conclusion will be disappointed. There's no silver lining. There is nothing up my sleeve. And although I've seen a lot of therapists, I do not claim to be one and thus cannot offer anything close to professional counseling advice. The truth is, I have lots of questions and few answers. I suppose the closest thing to a happy ending is that I've chosen to keep going. "Onwards we go." I believe that phrase should still pertain to me, and my future.

Grief continues to hound me. Grief's accomplices plague me: Anxiety. Disbelief. Sleep loss. Forgetfulness. Disconnection. Lack of focus. Avoidance. Loneliness. Anger. Sadness. Guilt. I still have to remind myself to take deep breaths. I still need exercise to stay a step ahead of a mood crash. I cry - a lot. I hurt. I suffer from breakdowns. I still fall down at the grocery store. The need to run away is still strong, and that devil is still on my shoulder, coaxing me into a tailspin in the midnights of my mind. I'm vulnerable and flawed, directionless and passionless. I still carry the guilt that I passed on the cancer gene to my son. I still can't always sleep through the entire night. Certain songs still shatter me. Above all else, I still pine for those days when Barb and I and Jasper were together... as a family. I miss that feeling of 'true happiness'. I'll never get to say: "My life is perfect" again. Honestly, sometimes I don't know what keeps me going.

It's Barb. I'm still in love with Barb. Thank God for Barb. I promised Jasper I'd take care of his mother and his dog. I seem to be fulfilling that promise – though at times I may be falling short of the mark. Barb and I are still in love. Despite the dismal odds of bereaved parents staying in a marriage, Barb and I have remained together. Sure, a lot of things have changed in the marriage. We give each other space when needed. She respects that I might need to run away for a time on my motorcycle.

She doesn't worry if she doesn't hear from me or I don't check in while I'm in isolation crossing the Valley of Fire or the Salt Flats. We respect each other's need to grieve, whatever form that might take. I've relied on Barb for so much and she's been very patient with me. We've worked together through some tough stuff. She has been so strong and so supportive of me. Of course, Barb struggles with grief too – but differently then I do. Just like Jasper, Barb has immersed herself in a wide variety of activities: everything from playing the drums to taking an off-road motorcycle course to hang gliding. She's always learning new skills and pushing her limits. She's currently taking a degree in songwriting. Several of her songs are outlets for her grief. They blow me away. I'm very proud of her and so fortunate to be able to call her my wife. So although we've lost our previous form as a 'family', and at times we struggle with the house full of empty rooms syndrome, we've chosen to keep going - together.

I still have my faith. Its different now though, like a veil has been lifted and I have a clearer understanding of it all. I think I've brought God down a couple of notches in my esteem. At one point a church minister told me I was stronger than some of the characters of the Old Testament, because many of them had denounced God. He himself was surprised I had not given up on God. I haven't, but I also don't have much to do with Him either. He's largely absent in my life lately. Maybe it's a faith of convenience. I'll call on Him when and if I need to. I do have some anger towards Him: sometimes I feel that this flesh and bone carcass cannot contain the rage and fire that I'd like to unleash on 'God's Plan'. I guess one reason I still consider myself a believer is the expectation that someday it will all be revealed to me as to why Jasper had to die. Despite my anger, and frustration and unanswered questions, I remain a believer. The existence of a 'Great Beyond' means Jasper is still out there in some form, and that gives me the hope that I'll see him again someday.

I still have so many questions. Why? Why did this happen to *my* family? What's next? Does anyone care? Will anyone remember Jasper? Did he just slip into the shadows and... he's gone? *So what* I've had this rich adventurous life: now what? Why go on? Should I give up? How do I go on? What do I do now? Do I pursue a new career? I'm open to learning. Open to trying things differently. It's hard to get excited about career aspirations though. My dream to build wooden boats is done.

Maybe I'll write another book? I may be fragile, frustrated, floundering and fucked up – but I can still alliterate. I've found writing to be cathartic. It organizes my thoughts and gets my history back in order in my head. Though, I'm certainly not healed just because I wrote a book. Writing my history reminds me of what a fantastic life I've had, and gives me reason to believe it could keep going that direction. It's just hard to keep writing this 'Great Adventure Story' when one of your main characters dies right in the middle.

The verdict is still out whether that 'Great Story' is a comedy or a tragedy. It definitely has its share of tragic events, but I haven't let them stop me from having a good laugh. I'm a Comedian. It's often to my detriment, as folks believe I must be doing okay because of the funny face I'm showing, when in fact I'm hurting on the inside. I'm a Magician. I can show you these lovely daffodils in one hand, all the while obscuring behind me my 'saw-trick-gone-wrong'. Upstage I'm attempting to pull a rabbit out of a hat, but behind the curtain, I'm in over my head, drowning in a Houdini Water Torture Cell trick. I don't mean to be glib. No one wants to see a clown when you've paid for a magic show. Is my story a comedy if I conclude the book with a good pun? Sometimes I can't help but think that someone, somewhere, is playing out a big joke at my expense. Is it all just a well-orchestrated illusion?

Someday, when the grand curtain is pulled back for me, I will be reunited with Jasper. I will hold him tightly again... and tell him I love him. I want to run my hands through his hair. Oh, to be playing together again. Misbehavin' together. Joking again. Lying on our backs taking in the magic of a night sky. Laughing. To swim in the sea again with him, drying our frigid bodies on the hot boards of the island's dock... and then the feel of the salt on the back of his neck. We'll snuggle on the couch with a bowl of popcorn. I'll intertwine his long fingers with mine. To watch those fingers dance across piano keys once again. I'll get to hear him chatter incessantly. Or we'll just sit and say nothing for hours on end, ignoring each other while we're both deep into our books. Nothing need be said. Oh, just to see his smile again... Jasper.

But until that day I will continue on. Jasper would want me to do that. If I were the one who died, wouldn't I want *him* to continue on? I'd want him to live the greatest life possible. My memories grow ever distant and fade to dreams as time marches on, and I am faced with a cold hard world in his absence. It's getting harder to recall him. He disappears. But I will continue on.

Again, I look back on that journal entry I made just previous to Jasper passing away. Oddly enough, even though I wrote it for him at the time, it now also applies to me in my current circumstances. It has such perfect sentiments that I can apply to myself now:

> Hope has fallen away. It lies in the muddy ditch by the roadside, trampled by the passing horses and carts. It is mangled and bent and cannot be reformed. But: "There is always Hope". Is there? I can only see one inevitable outcome. The way has been lost. I see it in your sunken hollow eyes and how you struggle to hold your head up. 'The Battle' is lost. It is over. And yet, 'The Fight' goes on around you. There is still a light in your eyes - a spark that could ignite a fire. So, something of you is still there. Knock off the heavy burden weighing down on your slouched shoulders. Get up. Keep going. Take up the broken piece of Hope by the side of the road. Force it and stretch it for all you are worth into a shining shield. Gather up your remaining strength and couple it to your Faith with Love. Make your last stand one to be remembered.

I *will* get up. I *will* keep going.

There is still a spark in me. I need to reform that broken shield. I still have my faith and I still am capable of love. My life is important. It's too valuable to just throw away, especially so being a cancer survivor, and being in a position where my time might be limited on this earth… well, if I'm a time bomb ticking, I'm going down kicking! And while I sometimes feel I'd like to follow Jasper immediately, I know deep down that I'm not done here yet. There's still work and a purpose for me here. There's still Hope.

§

July on the Oregon coast. The trailhead has a simple sign indicating the direction of the beach with an arrow, but no indication of how far it is. Barb and I follow a loose 'trail' that snakes around high, grass-covered dunes. The wind has carried drifts of sand over the route, obscuring sections and making it tricky to follow. The dunes are big enough that I can't see any further than the next mound of sand. There's an entire ocean out there somewhere in front of me, but I don't have any idea of how far away it is.

The sand is deep and it takes some effort to walk in. My boots sink into it with each footstep. The sun is intense. Only a few minutes into the trail and I'm hot and sweaty.

"I'm taking my boots off," I tell Barb. "Maybe it'll be easier in bare feet?"

Barb takes her footwear off too. The sand is burning hot. I look for tufts of grass on the edge of the trail to avoid the searing sand. There aren't too many opportunities for a step of respite from the burn.

Barb and I plod on together. I follow her around the base of a sandy hill only to be met by yet another dune. I think I can hear the faint roar of the surf now, but there's still no evidence of the ocean that lays somewhere beyond.

Barb seems to be doing so much better in this deep stuff than me. She's making progress skirting along the edge. I try to quicken my pace, but the sand holds me back.

"Do you think it's much further?" I ask. It's a rhetorical question. I'm looking for an exterior source of encouragement, as I'm starting to doubt whether I can do this. Maybe she's feeling like going back too? I slog onward.

"Geez, these dunes sure block the view and muffle all the sound." I'm whining.

We hike onwards. There's still no ocean around the next dune. This is beginning to feel too much like work. Is it really worth the effort? I don't actually voice them, but I have thoughts of doubt: "This sand is too tough to walk in with this heat. Who knows how far that beach could be yet? I've been walking a long time now. Maybe I should go back? Maybe I should give up?"

"No," I tell myself, "Jasper never gave up. Jasper would keep going. I'm going to keep going. He'd want to hike this through to the end. Onwards we go."

I find a new stride. The expectation and anticipation of seeing the ocean grows. I have a renewed strength.

"We must be getting close now," I say with hopefulness. "I think I can hear the surf!"

The path suddenly goes straight up the face of a dune. This looks hopeful. I crest the top.

"Wow."

There are no words. Nothing need be said between us.

From our vantage point high above the beach on the final dune, the coastline stretches off to an eternity in each direction. In front of me, the sky and sea fall away beyond the horizon. The sun is beaming gentle rays onto me. My feet are planted, half-buried into the cooler, grainy beach sand.

The wind is tugging at the shoreline grasses around me. It whips up the breaking surf, to hang in the air as a thin white mist down the length of the beach. The pounding Pacific sucks and pulls against the long low beach, the sound resonating in my ears. The singing gulls reel overhead in a dance. I can smell the salt, seaweed, and beach grass on the air. Everything is so vivid. I take a deep, deep breath. I feel alive. I am so happy that I kept going.

I take Barb's hand, and say with a smile, "Jasper would like this."

§

What it takes for me to overcome my suffering and crippling depression can be overwhelming. Regardless of that, Jasper would want me to keep living life to its fullest. Not just surviving, but living. Not just being alive, but feeling alive. I'm living for Jasper, embracing life again, as a testament to my love for him and his 'joie de vivre'.

EPILOGUE

I THINK I MISS YOU EVEN MORE

It's Friday afternoon. Four o'clock. He should be here any minute. I look up the hill of highway 101 for signs of the school bus. I'm waiting with Pippa outside the Lund Community Center. There's the bus. Pippa gets excited when I mention Jasper's name. As the bus pulls to a stop, I see him moving forward from the backseat, swaying under the weight of his heavy backpack. Four kids step off. There's the smile I love.

"Hi Papa!"

I get a big hug.

I lift his bag onto my shoulder. Pippa is jumping up and down and whining with joy at the sight of him. We slowly stroll down the curvy roadway, holding hands. Pippa has a new spring in her trot that was missing on our way up the hill. He talks and talks. Occasionally I get a word in and we laugh. We are on the final descent of the road down into Lund. It's a gorgeous sunny afternoon. The village is not overly busy, with only a few people about. The ocean below Lund is sparkling.

We need to make a decision. Should we go left to Nancy's Bakery and have a hot chocolate and a cinnamon bun? We usually save that for cold rainy Fridays. No, he decides, it's too nice a day to be inside. We stay on course for the Lund General Store. Pippa gets tied up outside. Once inside, we grab the usual Friday afternoon fare: a Jones soda each and a bag of Hawkin's Cheezies to share. He makes idle conversation with the checkout lady and makes her giggle.

We head back out into the sunshine. We crack open the sodas, but "save the Cheezies for the boat ride home, Papa." Tucked inside the bottle-caps are the usual ridiculous fortunes telling of how lucky we will be and how we will live a long and happy life.

We peruse the bulletin board outside the store for a few minutes. "That's a good price for firewood, Papa." He tears the phone number off the ad.

We head down the stairs to the back of the hotel. This is where the Lund Post Office is. I check the contents of our mailbox while he chats to Ruth, the Postmistress. They're like old friends. We leave her in stitches. We walk past the art gallery and down the ramp to our waiting runabout.

Pippa takes up her precarious position in the bow. It's a wonder she stays on the boat sometimes. Jasper unties the lines as I start the engine. We've got the routine down to an art. We don't even have to speak.

We point the boat in the direction of Sevilla Island and putt-putt slowly home. We're well into the Cheezies now. Jasper shares the especially odd-shaped freaky large ones with me. He complains I'm eating them all.

The ride is over in less than five minutes. We go through the opposite routine of shutting down the engine and tying up the boat. Jasper and Pippa sprint up the ramp to the house at the top of the dock and I follow behind with the empty soda bottles and his backpack.

"I'm going to start supper so it's ready when Mama gets home." I tell him.

"Oh C'mon Papa, let's go explore the beach."

I give in. I bring the Cheezies. Off we go, two boys and their dog exploring the rocky shore of an island, in the sunshine of a Friday afternoon. Just playing - as every boy should.

Then, off he goes around the point. Just out of my sight, just out of my reach.

Although I can no longer see him or touch him, I know that he is still there. And I know that eventually I will catch up to him... and we will laugh, and we will play, and we will eat Cheezies in the sun together again.

*Author's note: I can hear him critique this ending, and see him roll his eyes at me. "Oh, Papa... that is such a *Cheezie* ending." He always did like a good pun. He would also tell me to leave a few pages empty here at the end, because he wants me to explore the beach a bit further yet, before I follow him around the point...

(not) The End
Onwards we go...

NOTES

ACKNOWLEDGEMENTS

For additional content visit:

www.onwardswego.ca

Jasper was a big advocate for donating blood. If you are able, donate to a blood bank.

I wish to acknowledge all the families currently going through a similar plight to what we faced. Right now there are babies, children and teens fighting for their lives against cancer. Learn more about childhood cancers and how you can make a difference here:

www.thetruth365.org

WITH THANKS

Barbra. I would not be in this world today were it not for your unbound love and friendship.

Ronald McDonald House British Columbia for providing us with a home away from home. It is indeed 'a house that love built' and I will forever treasure the friendships that were founded there.

The Doctors and Nurses of the British Columbia Children's Hospital and the Canuck Place Children's Hospice for going above and beyond.

Rick and the staff of the Cowichan Valley Hospice Society for piecing 'Humpty Dumpty' back together again.

Lorne at Avid Fitness and Frank at Suncoast Cycles for getting me 'back in the saddle'.

Chelsey Whittle for the use of her eloquent quote.

Lesley Marijke McCandless for taking the time to offer her expertise and experience as an editor.

Chad, and my circle of friends, who so patiently put up with me and continually show me their unconditional love.

Barb's family for their continued love and support.

Thank you to everyone that supported Barb and Jasper and I through prayers, thoughts, funds or gifts during our journey. We truly felt your care and love.

REFERENCES

Grahame, K., & Shepard, E. H. (1983). The Wind In The Willows. New York: Scribner

Hemingway, Ernest (2006). The Sun Also Rises. New York: Scribner

Housman, A.E. (1896). A Shropshire Lad. London: K. Paul, Trench, Treubner

CPSIA information can be obtained
at www.ICGtesting.com
Printed in the USA
LVOW12s1725290318
571634LV00003B/692/P